I0440540

MAGICAL APPLE CIDER VINEGAR

V. GANGAN

Angan Publications Ltd,

707B Richardson Road,

Hillsborough, Auckland, New Zealand 1042

Fist printing 2014

10 9 8 7 6 5 4 3 2 1

ISBN: 149923662X
ISBN-13: 978-1499236620

DEDICATION

Dedicated to my wife.

CONTENTS

ACKNOWLEDGMENTS

This book acknowledges the hundreds of researchers, scientists, academicians and writers, who have kept the fire alive in the miniscule literature that exists about the benefits of apple cider vinegar.

i

PRAISE FOR APPLE CIDER VINEGAR

"Apple cider vinegar is the icing on the cake. I had always heard about apple cider vinegar. Everyone in the world should be drinking this on a daily basis!" **Dr. Steven Gibb**

***

"If your skin is problematic or you're having a lot of breakouts, (apple cider vinegar) is really healing. It's a little bit stinky but if you're not sleeping over at your boyfriend's, it's really effective."

Hollywood actor Scarlett Johansson

***

"I drink a tall glass of water with lemon juice, ACV, and organic honey in the morning, instead of coffee and can truly see and feel the difference in my health." **Tessa Dunn, California City, USA**

"I did the ACV/honey diet several years ago and I noticed after a time that I had lost my cravings for sweets (and I had a real sweet tooth!)." **Jerri, USA**

***

"ACV works fast for me. I had digestive problems for three years. Now my heartburn is gone. Also tingle in my calf and toes is gone because of ACV. Cider vinegar helped me get off drugs and pass my drug test for THC (cannabis or marijuana). I have been drug free since 2003. I wish to keep using it for health." **Grant, USA**

***

"Apple cider vinegar really helps. I have been using it for four months. I feel great; I lost weight, and I have no more issues of constipation, sinus or acne. I feel young. I love my body." **Shelby, USA**

***

PRAISE FOR THIS BOOK ON AMAZON

"This book is very good for detailing the amazing benefits of apple cider vinegar. I would recommend." **Judy Vinals, USA**

***

"This contained the information I needed to know about apple cider. Great read if (you) are looking to add apple cider vinegar to your diet." **Lydia, USA**

***

PRAISE FOR THE AUTHOR

"You are just awesome! Thank you so much for all of your replies. Thank you for all of your willingness to help us (by) answering our questions. I am truly glad I have found your articles. I will definitely encourage my family and friends to try ACV as it has just helped me beyond what I expected. Thank you. Thank you. Thank you! God bless you." **Chrey, USA**

***

THE ELIXIR

The father of medicine, Hippocrates, used it as an elixir.

On his ambitious voyages, sailor Columbus carried apple cider vinegar to cure scurvy.

The Bible has reference to vinegar. ("When Jesus therefore had received the vinegar, he said, It is finished: and he bowed his head, and gave up the ghost." John 19:30.)

American actress and singer Hilary Duff uses it to treat pimples.

Meet magical apple cider vinegar, the natural remedy for many modern ailments.

1. MY EXPERIENCE WITH ACV

Many years ago, I was introduced to the benefits of apple cider vinegar by a friend, who mentioned it as a dietary supplement.

A few years passed. As my interest in healthy living grew, I came across an article about the health benefits of apple cider vinegar, and I remembered my friend. I freshly began my research and was very surprised by the variety of benefits offered by Apple Cider Vinegar (ACV).

I got curious and set up to do further research. Since Internet did not have much information about apple cider vinegar, I bought books on ACV and read voraciously. I bought a bottle of organic apple cider vinegar, and began using it at home. Being a skeptic, I started by drinking ACV once a day.

Initially I did not like the taste; soon I discovered a trick to get over the strong smell of ACV (which I will describe later in the book). Then I introduced ACV to salad dressings, much to the dismay of my family. I began to feel more energetic.

Soon, cider vinegar found its way from kitchen to bathroom. At home, I have used vinegar as a deodorizer, skin cleanser, mouthwash, hair conditioner and muscle relaxant. Sharing my experience was the natural next step for me. I began writing articles and posting links on social networks. The more I wrote, the more I got comments and questions. I researched more and answered those questions.

Then one commenter asked whether I had a reference book or handbook about apple cider vinegar. I had read many books, but there wasn't a single book that was brief, easy-to-understand, and included practical tips.

I realized that I had written articles about ACV, answered people's queries, and now it was important to put together a book that could be used as a guide for getting the most health benefits from the use of apple cider vinegar.

I began writing this book. The next challenge was to keep the book concise for a busy exccutive or at-home mother, who could read the book in a day, and begin using apple cider vinegar right away. This became a challenge as I tried to include everything I knew.

The next stage was to trim down the book and focus on the most important issues. Here I relied on feedback from the readers of my website. I got most queries from readers about three issues - how to lose weight, improve hair quality, and get healthy skin with apple cider vinegar. So I decided to focus mainly on those three ailments, while briefly delving into other important uses of cider vinegar.

That's how this book was born. In this revised edition of the book, I have added a chapter dedicated to answering the most common questions I usually receive about using apple cider vinegar. If you are in a hurry, head straight to the Frequently Asked Questions chapter at the end of this book, where you will find most of your queries answered. Alternatively you can directly go to the chapters relevant to the health issue you are facing and find a solution there.

I am very pleased to put this book in your hands, and hope it will be a worthy companion on your journey towards good health. If you have any questions, feel free to email me via my website: www.101WaysToLife.com

V. Gangan
Auckland, New Zealand
2014

2. ABOUT APPLES

An apple a day keeps doctor away. This proverb has become popular for a good reason. Apples are available in most parts of the world, and are a rich source of nutrients essential for complete wellbeing.

Apples are known to reduce the risks of life-threatening chronic diseases including:

- cardiovascular diseases
- high blood pressure
- diabetes

The key components found in apples - polyphenols and fiber - are responsible for reducing the risk of these diseases. A 2014 report entitled, "*Diet-Microbe Interactions in the Gut*"[1] looked at, among other things, various studies investigating the impact of apples on cardio-metabolic disease risk factors and possible mechanisms linked to the gut microbiota. The report noted that the consumption of apples has been associated with "beneficial lipid changes, delayed glucose response, antioxidative and anti-inflammatory properties, reduced blood pressure and effects on gut microbiota composition."

Also, apples have properties that can reduce the risk of tumor and cancer. In a 2014 report entitled "*Apple Polyphenols in Cancer Prevention*",[2] researchers have found that apple procyanidins possess many physiological functions such as anti-oxidative and anti-tumor activities.

Apples: A Source of Anti-oxidants

To understand how apples provide essential anti-oxidants, let us first understand oxidation.

Oxidation is a natural process that is taking place all around us. When you leave a slice of apple on the table for a while, it turns brown because of oxidation. Similarly, if you happen to cut your skin while peeling an apple, the blood flowing out of the wound soon becomes thick and black, and forms a protective layer on the cut. That's oxidation.

In short, oxidation uses oxygen in the air and changes the properties of a cell in human body, fruits, vegetables and even fish. While oxidation is mostly good, occasionally it goes wrong and produces damaged cells, known as 'free radicals'. These 'free radicals' are also produced by air pollution, smoking and even alcohol consumption. Even physical exercise produces free radicals in the body.

These free radicals then attack other, good cells, leaving

them injured. This causes the DNA of the injured cell to change. The injured cell now becomes the new 'free radical', and this chain reaction rapidly spreads to other good cells, leading to the creation of a whole army of free radicals.

While human body has an in-built mechanism to fight free radicals, modern life exposes us to an onslaught of free radicals, which soon get out of control and cause a disease. This is why oxidation is one of the causes of chronic and degenerative diseases like cancer, heart disease and neuronal degeneration.

So how do you protect yourself from the harm caused by these free radicals? With the help of anti-oxidants. The most familiar anti-oxidants are vitamin C, vitamin E, beta-carotene and minerals selenium and manganese. Lesser-known but important anti-oxidants are flavonoids (the largest group of anti-oxidants) and polyphenols.

The USDA (the United States Department of Agriculture) recommends fruits and vegetables as a source of anti-oxidants to help fight these free radicals. Anti-oxidants found in apples and other fruits, nuts, vegetables, whole grains and legumes either stop the chain reaction caused by free radicals or prevent it completely. Apples are the most important source of anti-oxidants. In fact, a list released by the USDA has put apples among the top sources of antioxidants.[3]

When the USDA ranked 275 selected foods based on anti-oxidant value per serving, apples, rather 'Red Delicious' brand of apples (with skin), found a spot among the top three foods. It is worth noting that anti-oxidant value of apples is greatly reduced if the skin is removed. As such, eat apples with skin. Make sure that you have washed them thoroughly so as to remove the remnants of pesticides from apple skin. To do this, put a few drops of white vinegar in a bowl of filtered water and rinse apples thoroughly. White vinegar is very effective in removing pesticides from fruits and vegetables.

In the USDA list, the Red Delicious brand of apples is followed by Granny Smith apples, and then Gala apples for their anti-oxidant value. That's right - not all apples are created equal. Researchers believe that certain varieties of apples offer more health benefits. One such study found that the U.S.-produced apples, particularly 'Delicious', had some superior quality characteristics compared to fruit from other origins.[4]

It is therefore important to choose quality apples. Choosing organic apples is logical for two reasons: the origin of apples is known; and organic apples are free of chemicals and pesticides.

No matter which brand of apples you choose, it is important to make apples a part of your daily diet.

Apples provide protection against many illnesses, such as:

- Parkinson's
- Alzheimer's
- Diabetes

- Heart-related diseases
- Irritable bowel syndrome
- Hemorrhoids
- Gallstones
- Cancer
- Cataract
- Digestion-related issues including diarrhea and constipation
- Liver-related illnesses

By now you may wonder: if fruits and vegetables are so effective in preventing illnesses, why are they not prescribed by doctors? There are many reasons. When we consult a doctor or are admitted to the hospital, it is usually too late for natural remedies to be effective; the urgent need is to cure the illness, which is possible with medical intervention.

The second reason is our attitude. We live in the era of immediate gratification; we hit the 'back' button on web browser if a webpage is slow to load; we seek refund if the pizza is delivered late. When we fall sick, we seek immediate relief with medicines.

Third and most important, natural medicines cannot be patented, and therefore, there's no profit to be made from them. On the other hand, prescription drugs are not only profitable to sell but also are very expensive to produce, because of the extensive research and development required to invent them.

On an average, it takes 14 years of research to invent one drug. According to a study by the *Forbes magazine*,[5] pharmaceutical companies spend about $5 billion for developing and testing a new drug. This shows that there's a commercial benefit to sell these drugs.

However, here's a less acknowledged fact: these drugs are literally killing us. According to one study,[6] drugs prescribed in hospitals are now the fourth largest cause of deaths in the United States - more than the number of fatalities in vehicle accidents.

I am not against medicines. In fact, I believe that medicines are a life-saving intervention. Drugs are essential to save the situation brought about by chronic neglect of body caused by lack of nutritional diet or exercise. However, allopathic medicine should be used in situations that cannot be reversed easily.

These drugs therefore must complement natural remedies. For this reason, I like the phrase *'complementary medicine'* rather than *'alternative medicine'* for natural cures. Using natural remedies on a regular basis will help reduce the need for frequent and extensive medical intervention. The best approach is to follow a nutritional diet on a daily basis, so that the need to see a doctor or seek medical intervention is reduced.

I strongly urge you to make apples and other fruits and vegetables a part of your everyday food.

3. ABOUT ACV

Apple cider vinegar is also known as cider vinegar, Vinagre de Manzana, Vinagre de Sidra de Manzana, and Vinaigre de Cidre. Its scientific name is Malus sylvestris, and it is from the family of Rosaceae.

Vinegar is wine gone sour. In fact, that's how vinegar was discovered - a cask of expired wine fermented and became sour. The word vinegar originated from Latin words: '*vinum*' for wine, and '*acer*' for sharp, and French words: '*vin*' for wine and '*aigre*' for sour. Thus, *vinaigre* means sour wine.

Vinegar is the next stage in winemaking. In fact, vinegar is made by fermenting alcoholic liquids. It mainly contains water and acetic acid (the chemical formula is CH_3COOH).

Many centuries ago, vinegar found its use as an industrial cleaner because of its acid-like qualities. Only later did vinegar find a spot in cooking and diet. Different types of vinegar are produced from a range of sources including kiwifruits, coconuts, palm, dates, barley, apples, sugarcane, grapes, rice, wheat, millet, wine and beer.

The acetic acid bacteria cause apple juice to become vinegar during fermentation. Vinegar can be made in a traditional way using slow fermentation, or can be mass produced using fast fermentation.

The natural fermentation can take months. To speed up the process, the 'mother' of vinegar (which is culture bacteria) is added during fermentation, and then oxygen is added using a pump system or turbine. This fermentation and oxygenation first coverts fruit sugars to alcohol, and alcohol to vinegar.

Such fast fermentation takes two to three days to produce vinegar. For the modern age, apple cider vinegar was one of the most hidden types of vinegars until it came back to limelight, thanks to endorsements from Hollywood celebrities like Scarlett Johansson who uses apple cider vinegar for maintaining glowing skin.

4. HOW COMMERCIAL ACV IS MADE

Apple cider vinegar is made from apple must; whole apples (including skin and core) are crushed using thousands of pounds of weight to obtain apple must.

Methods used for commercially making apple cider vinegar differ from brand to brand. For winemakers, producing vinegar is the easy part, making wine isn't. Which prompted celebrated winemaker August Sebastiani to say, "God wants to make vinegar, and we have to stop Him!"

Micro-organisms convert fruit sugar to vinegar in two stages. The first stage is alcoholic fermentation using yeast (a type of fungus) to convert natural sugars into alcohol. The second is acid fermentation using micro-organism acetobacter to change the alcohol to acetic acid. (Later in the book, I'll discuss how to make ACV at home.)

5. LOSING WEIGHT WITH ACV

Using apple cider vinegar for weight loss and good health is not a new trend, though it is gaining popularity like a fad, and for good reasons.

How Does It Work

Apple cider vinegar has found a secure spot in the kitchen since time immemorial.

ACV is used for everything from boosting immune system to treating digestion problems, lowering blood pressure, removing warts, and the most popular use of cider vinegar – weight loss. Limited research exists to show exactly how apple cider vinegar works for weight loss, though extensive research material is available about the properties of apple.

A few theories explain how our body benefits from apple cider vinegar's weight loss properties.

In a 2009 study published in the *Bioscience, Biotechnology, and Biochemistry Journal*,[7] researchers studied the effects of acetic acid, the main component of apple cider vinegar, on the reduction of body fat mass in obese Japanese people.

The subjects were randomly assigned to three groups of similar body weight, body mass index (BMI), and waist circumference. Researchers conducted a 12-week double-blind trial, which meant neither the participants nor researchers knew which group was control group and which one was test group. Participants in each group consumed 500 ml of a beverage every day, containing either 15 ml of vinegar (750 mg acetic acid or AcOH), 30 ml of vinegar (1,500 mg AcOH), or 0 ml of vinegar (0 mg AcOH, as placebo effect).

Researchers found that both the vinegar-drinking groups showed significant reduction in body weight, BMI, visceral fat area, waist circumference, and serum triglyceride levels, compared to the placebo group.

The study concluded that daily intake of vinegar might be useful in the prevention of metabolic syndrome by reducing obesity. ACV also contains enzymes that increase metabolism rate in our body. A higher metabolism boosts the speed of burning fat.

Some studies have found that cider vinegar helps in lowering cholesterol. In a 2008 study published in the *Pakistan Journal of Biological Sciences*,[8] researchers fed apple cider vinegar (6% w/w) diet to two groups - normal rats and diabetic rats - for four weeks.

They monitored fasting blood glucose, glycated haemoglobin and lipid profile of both the groups. Scientists noted significant reduction of LDL cholesterol and significant increase of HDL cholesterol (good cholesterol) in normal rats. Apple cider vinegar also reduced serum triglyceride and increased HDL cholesterol in diabetic animals.

Researchers concluded that apple cider vinegar improved the serum lipid profile in normal and diabetic rats by decreasing serum triglyceride, LDL cholesterol and increasing serum HDL cholesterol, and may be of great value in managing the diabetic complications.

Similarly, the fibers in ACV cause a feeling of fullness sooner, even with less food eaten. Fibers also have one more important role in weight loss – that of detoxification. Fibers absorb excess fat and toxins, which are then removed from our body through urine. This is one of the reasons why frequent visits to toilet are common during the first stage of an ACV diet.

ACV also improves digestive system, and regularizes bowel movements. Healthy digestion system makes it easier for body to extract nutrients from food, and remove accumulated fat and toxins.

Additionally, cider vinegar lowers blood sugar level. As a result, the body makes less insulin. Extensive medical studies show that lowering the levels of insulin causes weight loss. These factors collectively contribute to weight loss and burning off excess fat. Irrespective of the exact science behind apple cider vinegar, there is anecdotal evidence of people losing weight successfully by drinking apple cider vinegar regularly. Losing weight is possible if correct approach is followed for drinking ACV. Let us see the right way of introducing an ACV diet.

6. DRINKING ACV THE RIGHT WAY

On your weight loss journey it is important to remember that losing weight is not a destination or the ultimate goal. It's a journey. And it needs commitment, because it is an ongoing effort that becomes a second nature through regular practice. ACV only makes that journey easier and accelerates progress.

To get the most benefit out of cider vinegar, follow a routine for drinking it. The right way to drink ACV:

- Dilute it
- Drink daily, twice a day
- Drink at the right time
- Drink in small quantity

For best results, you need to drink ACV regularly. And it's not very difficult if you follow the tip here. You only need to drink a small quantity. The hard part is to remember to drink it every day. And drink it at the right time every day. The tip is to carry your ACV drink bottle around and keep sipping the drink throughout the day.

ACV needs to be had in moderation. Increasing the quantity of ACV is not going to speed up your weight loss, and could even be detrimental to your health. Read the chapter "*Side Effects of ACV*" later in the book.

The best time to drink apple cider vinegar is an hour or so before the meal. I prefer to drink apple cider vinegar immediately after waking up or soon after my morning tea. That way, I remember to drink it every morning. And I drink the second glass of ACV in the evening, about an hour before dinner. This helps in clearing up my stomach for the meal. I try to eat dinner early – at least three hours before going to bed.

Based on feedback from many of my readers, I gather that it is a common practice to make one liter of ACV drink in the morning, fill it up in a bottle, take it along to work, and drink it during the day as mentioned earlier.

Now let's see how to make the ACV drink.

7. MAKING ACV DRINK

Apple Cider Vinegar is acidic. It contains 5% acetic acid. This is why cider vinegar drink is made by diluting it with water. Don't drink it neat or straight from the bottle as some people I know do this.

Put two to three teaspoons of ACV in a glass of water (16 ounces, 250 ml), and drink. You may be tempted to put more ACV in water, but that will be futile as this is unlikely to give more health benefits. Also, ACV has a strong smell. So you wouldn't want to make a strong drink. To get rid of the smell, here's a trick I discovered by accident.

When I began drinking ACV, I did not like the smell. Then one freezing, winter night, I warmed water and put ACV in it. That's when I realized that the ACV odor is not very strong when it is consumed in lukewarm water. Try it. However, do this when absolutely necessary; excessive heat may destroy the nutritional value of cider vinegar. It sensitivity to ultra-violet rays. If you are going out in the sun after applying apple cider vinegar, please use a good sunscreen lotion, so as to avoid any harmful effect of UV rays. This is another reason why apple cider vinegar should be applied on skin at night, instead of during the day.

Is ACV Suitable For Your Skin?

ACV is safe for use on skin. As it balances the pH factor of the skin, most people find ACV very refreshing. If you cannot tolerate the smell, you can do one or more of these things:

- Apply less frequently
- Dilute ACV with more water
- Wash off ACV after five to 10 minutes

You may be one of the few people with sensitive skin. ACV may cause skin reaction even in highly diluted form. If this happens, stop using it, and look for another remedy for acne.

is also likely that you may not like the taste of ACV initially. To improve the taste, put a teaspoon of organic honey in it.

Adding honey to ACV has two advantages – it improves the flavor of the drink, and it also compounds the health benefits of the drink. Honey is known for its antibacterial properties, and is also a good source of minerals including potassium, magnesium, calcium, iron, phosphate, sodium chloride and sulphur. Some types of honey also contain many vitamins. The best honey I have had is Manuka honey, found in New Zealand (where I live).

To make ACV routine more enjoyable, add it to your tea. The method is simple – add boiling water to tea leaves or tea bag, honey or maple syrup. Once the tea is brewed to your satisfaction, drop two teaspoons of cider vinegar. I prefer the pure Canadian maple syrup, not the sugary syrup.

Alternatively mix it with coffee, though that is not my preference. Mixing ACV with caffeine is not advisable – caffeine dehydrates the body and increases blood pressure – which is opposite of what apple cider vinegar is expected to do. Similarly, it is recommended to avoid mixing ACV with cola or aerated drinks, and certainly not with hard liquor.

Apple Cider Vinegar Is A Habit

One of the common questions I get is – how long does it take to lose weight using apple cider vinegar diet?

Apple cider vinegar is not for people in a hurry to lose weight fast, though it is possible to lose weight quickly with apple cider vinegar, as I will explain later in the book.

As a natural product, apple cider vinegar offers a good alternative to other medicines for weight loss. But you shouldn't expect overnight results. Good things come to those who wait. Apple cider vinegar helps you reduce weight in a gradual fashion. Since apple cider vinegar offers so many benefits in addition to weight loss, it is not only acceptable but also advisable to make apple cider vinegar a part of your everyday diet. If you are looking for immediate weight loss, keep reading as I will share a plan to burn fat fast with ACV.

There's limited research to indicate how long it takes to lose weight with apple cider vinegar. Also, each person's body type is different. There are so many factors that influence weight loss – blood type, blood sugar levels, level of physical stamina and strength, genetics and any existing health conditions.

Based on anecdotal feedback received in response to my articles about cider vinegar, I can say that many have lost 10 to 15 pounds (about 6 to 9 kilos) in a few months, whereas some dieters have achieved the same goal in half of that time. Many motivated people have even lost five founds in a month. Weight loss with apple cider vinegar may take longer for some people. You too can lose weight if you are consistent and disciplined in drinking ACV. The ultimate responsibility of shedding extra pounds and getting back in shape rests with you. And it is never too late to begin – no matter what age or size you are.

8. BUYING THE RIGHT ACV

Not all vinegars are created equal. Which is why the success of your weight loss plan will depend on choosing the right vinegar. There are no cutting corners when it comes to buying your first bottle of cider vinegar. Good vinegar is not necessarily the most expensive on the shelf. Neither is it the cheapest.

To help you choose the right apple cider vinegar, I'll explain different types of cider vinegars available in the market.

White Vinegar

This is the most known and commonly found vinegar in the market. You will find this in your kitchen.

While white vinegar has multiple uses, it is completely irrelevant for the health benefits described in this book.

It doesn't contain the enzymes you will need to lose weight. If you have already bought this vinegar, use it in the kitchen.

Apple Cider Vinegar

This is the vinegar you need for your wellbeing. However, here too, the choice isn't simple. Many types of apple cider vinegar are available in the market.

To make it easier to decide, look for the following criteria in apple cider vinegar. If the cider vinegar you are buying passes the following test, then you have bought the correct vinegar.

Is it unfiltered?

Make sure you are buying unfiltered vinegar. When ACV is filtered, it will remove the mother of cider vinegar, and will be of no use for its health benefits.

Is it unpasteurized?

While making juices, the liquid is usually heated to kill harmful bacteria. This heating is called pasteurization. Unfortunately, the heating process cannot be applied selectively to just bad bacteria, and save good bacteria. As such, pasteurization removes nutrients and enzymes that give us the value we are looking for.

So look for apple cider vinegar that's unpasteurized and unfiltered. Additionally, if the cider vinegar is also made from organic apples, then you are in for a really good vinegar. Organic vinegar is free from harmful chemicals and pesticides.

Many brands in the market are mass-produced and fast-produced, by speeding up the fermentation process. You will need to buy a brand that's naturally and organically produced.

When it comes to buying apple cider vinegar, don't go by the looks. The healthiest apple cider vinegar is usually not the best-looking vinegar. In fact, a good bottle of cider vinegar is not very appealing to the eye – the liquid is pale in color, with floating elements of muddy 'mother' (which is bacterial culture) at the bottom.

Most good brands of apple cider vinegar are everlasting - they don't come with an expiry date. Good apple cider vinegar can be stored for a long time. In fact, vinegar is like wine - older the better.

The good brands of apple cider vinegar are: Bragg, Fleischmann, Dynamic Health and Vitacost. (Disclaimer: The author is not associated with any of these brands.)

Bragg Organic Apple Cider Vinegar

Advisor to Olympians, Dr Paul C. Bragg pioneered healthy lifestyle in the US, and set up a company that now makes apple cider vinegar. His daughter and nutritionist Patricia Bragg joined him in their venture to bring good health to people. The California-based company makes Bragg Organic Apple Cider Vinegar in wooden barrels.

The apple cider vinegar is reportedly made from organic apples, and is unfiltered, unheated and unpasteurized. It contains 5% acidity. The vinegar has the 'mother', which is a strand-like substance (enzymes) of protein molecules – this is where the health benefits of ACV are stored. Bragg and apple cider vinegar are almost synonymous in the United States.

You can request a free sample of Bragg Apple Cider Vinegar through their website.

Fleischmann

Fleischmann specializes in vinegars. This is probably one of the most expensive cider vinegars you will find. They have an interesting story. Back in the 1920s, Fleischmann wanted to make use of the alcohol that was a by-product of the bakers' yeast growth. So they began to make vinegars. That's how this California-based company entered the vinegar market.

Of course, after a few decades, when technology advanced, this by-product became less available. But the vinegars had become popular. So Fleischmann entered the specialty vinegar business. There is nothing to suggest that the comparatively higher price you pay for Fleischmann's cider vinegar is essentially ensuring a better product for you.

Dynamic Health

Founded in 1994, Dynamic Health is a relatively new name in the apple cider vinegar category, but sells value-for-money products. It makes apple cider vinegar from USDA certified organic apples. Dynamic Health offers the cheapest organic, unfiltered, unpasteurized apple cider vinegar. Interestingly, you will find Vitacost website sells all these brands.

Vitacost

Vitacost is known for health products and supplements. Its apple cider vinegar is made from organic apples in an unpasteurized way. It does not contain artificial sweeteners or coloring.

Vitacost products are price competitive, and depending on which country you are in, Vitacost vinegar may be marginally cheaper than Bragg. These are the top brands of apple cider vinegar to consider. No matter which brand you choose, buy a small bottle first and try it out. If you don't like the taste, you can change the brand, or buy pills of apple cider vinegar.

Liquid or Pills?

Apple cider vinegar is available in liquid as well as pills form. If you find the smell and taste of apple cider vinegar drink too strong, you may consider taking ACV pills. ACV pills are advertised to contain all the benefits of liquid ACV.

Unfortunately, it is not always possible to know the exact ingredients in ACV pills, which makes it difficult to form guidelines about how many pills to consume.

Usually, the options in the market may contain 285 mg or 500 mg pills. Each pill may have 35% acidic content, and is consumed before each meal. Because it is hard to verify the validity of claims made by these pill-makers, it is advisable to talk to a trusted local pharmacist. Personally, I haven't tried ACV pills.

Now that you know the good brands of ACV, let's also look at making your own cider vinegar at home.

9. MAKING ACV AT HOME

It is possible to make apple cider vinegar at home; the process is very easy. Because apple cider vinegar is made by fermentation and oxygenation, you need ideal temperature and storage conditions.

If these conditions are not right, apple cider vinegar may not form correctly. Worse still, it may breed harmful bacteria. As such, your first option should be to buy apple cider vinegar from the market.

If this is not possible, you can make apple cider vinegar at home. Even then, you should buy your first apple cider vinegar from the market. This will familiarize you with the taste of good apple cider vinegar; when you make ACV at home, you will know whether the ACV has fermented properly.

Of course, if you can make apple cider vinegar at home, you will have better control on ingredients, and you can be sure that your cider vinegar is organic and well-fermented. You should aim to make cider vinegar in November or December (in the Northern Hemisphere), because you need winter or fall variety of apples. Summer apples don't have enough sugar and are not suitable for making cider vinegar.

You will need to take apple "must" through fermentation and oxygenation stages to make good ACV.

There are four steps to making ACV:

- Apple must
- Yeast fermentation
- Acetic acid fermentation
- Clarification

1. Apple must

First, you may either grow organic apples in you backyard or buy certified organic apples from the market. While organic apples are free of pesticides, it is advisable to wash them thoroughly before use. I usually put a few teaspoons of white vinegar in a bowl of water and wash apples in the bowl.

Now, crush whole apples including the skin, seeds and stem. Some people prefer to remove seeds, as they fear arsenic contamination. Strain the juice and put it in a glass jar with wide mouth. This is where you need to add yeast to speed up fermentation. You can skip this step, but fermentation will take longer without yeast.

Don't buy the yeast used in bread-making. You need yeast that's used for beer-making. Mix only a small quantity of yeast in the juice.

2. Yeast fermentation

There are two stages to fermentation – yeast fermentation which takes about a month, and acetic fermentation which takes about two weeks. Yeast fermentation is the process where fruit sugar turns into alcohol. For this, fill the container to about 3 quarters and stir it every day. Fermentation will take about a month.

Important:

- Use only clean and dry spoon for stirring. If the spoon is wet or dirty, it may introduce undesirable bacteria and spoil your efforts.
- Avoid direct sunlight

3. Acetic acid fermentation

Once yeast fermentation is complete, wait for another week or two. This will allow the alcohol to covert to acetic acid.

4. Clarification

Now that acetic acid is formed in the jar, clarify the acetic acid so that no further fermentation is possible. For this you will need a cheesecloth or coffee filter. Filter the cider vinegar a few times.

This is the vinegar that you have worked so hard to make – your own organic apple cider vinegar.

Things to remember while making ACV at home:

- Keep the liquid away from sunlight. Even after ACV is ready, store it away from sunlight.

- Remember to stir the liquid every day. This one action I have found difficult to remember. Solution? Put a reminder on your smart-phone. It also helps to keep the jar in sight so that you remember to stir it when you visit the kitchen. If you don't stir it every day, it will not get sufficient oxygen, and the process of oxygenation will not take place.

- For making apple cider vinegar, maintain ideal temperature which is about 60 to 80 degrees Fahrenheit. If you don't have this temperature, then fermentation will be difficult.

- Because of the acetic content of cider vinegar, avoid metal container for making as well as storing vinegar. Use only glass, plastic, wood, enamel or stainless steel containers. I try to avoid plastic too.

- Apple cider vinegar doesn't have an expiry date. As long as it is stored away from sunlight, it could last for months.

10. LOSING WEIGHT FAST WITH ACV

Many people want to lose weight but they want to do it fast. Weight-watchers are usually in a hurry to shed extra pounds - they want to look attractive in a bikini as the summer approaches; or they want to go on a date; a prom night to attend; or they are getting married and want to look fabulous in the wedding gown; or they are just sick of feeling sick all the time, and want to take charge of their life.

Whatever your reason, remember - weight loss takes time. Rather, it should take time. Losing weight too quickly is not only unhealthy but could be dangerous too. Shedding too many kilos in a short time can put pressure on your heart. Also, a fast weight loss plan may make you look older, though thinner.

However, it is possible to lose weight in a healthy way with apple cider vinegar.

So what do you need to do?

First, keep drinking apple cider vinegar twice a day before meals, as usual. This will keep your metabolism rate high, make you fill full, and remove toxins from your body. You will then need to supplement your ACV diet with a healthy lifestyle. In other words, you can't expect miracles from ACV if you continue to eat junk food and lead a sedentary lifestyle.

Weight loss is a joint responsibility – you need to be committed to your weight loss goal, and do as much work externally as ACV is doing internally. Of course, I am not expecting you to make a drastic change in diet. But you will need to bring discipline in your diet as well as routine. (Yes, you should have a routine.)

Speed Up Your Weight Loss

Follow a few rules while you are on apple cider vinegar diet for weight loss. Let these rules become habits. These choices will not only help in weight loss but will also support overall health.

Stop junk

Avoid fatty food. Most fast food is fattening. Avoid deep-fried, highly saturated food. Also stay away from food containing too much salt or refined sugar. Sugar in its natural form (as found in fruits) is fine to consume. You may take a monthly 'diet holiday', when you satisfy your craving for fast food, desserts and alcohol for an entire day. On other days of the month, avoid junk food.

Begin periodic fasting

Take a monthly break from food for a day. Don't eat any food at all, even if it is healthy food. Just consume apple cider vinegar drink with honey twice. If such fasting is difficult, you may eat some fruit. Fasting helps vital organs in your body to rest and recover. These organs are - bladder, intestine, kidney and lever. They deserve rest.

The second benefit of fasting is the detox effect. Apple cider vinegar gets complete control of your body for a day, and it can work best with such monopoly over your body. Once you get used to the monthly fasting habit, you may increase the frequency to fortnightly and then to weekly fasting. You will be amazed how re-energized you will feel after the detoxification.

Start exercising

Losing weight is a two-sided coin - diet and exercise are the two sides. Imagine standing in front of a water tank. You are given the task of emptying the tank. There's a tap at the top that feeds water to the tank regularly, and there's another tap at the bottom that removes water from the tank. Both the taps are open. What's the fastest way to empty that tank? You are right - you need to turn off the feeding tap and you need to keep open the outlet tap.

Weight loss effort is pretty much the same - while you regulate the new calories entering your body, you need to find a way to burn existing calories, and that is why exercising is important. I am not suggesting marathon running or heavy weightlifting. If you have never or rarely worked out before, take baby steps. Begin with a leisurely walk around the block. Do it every day. After a week, try to increase the distance walked by about 50%. If you walked a mile in the first week, increase the distance to 1.5 miles in the second week. Also, increase walking speed. Once you get comfortable with the new distance and speed, introduce a small sprint in the middle of the walk.

Aim to increase duration to 40 minutes a day, five days a week. Here's an important point - ACV and exercise are complementary. Regular exercise coupled with ACV drinking every day will have a compounding effect on metabolism rate and weight loss.

Consider this. Metabolism rate is like the fuel efficiency of a car. Think of two cars - one with high fuel efficiency and the other with low. Take a 10-mile trip in each car. Note the amount of fuel consumed.

Less fuel-efficient car will consume more fuel for the same distance compared to the highly efficient car. Similarly, if you exercise regularly, you will have higher metabolism, which means, your body will burn more fat. And since ACV too helps in improving metabolism, you will get more health benefit for the same distance walked compared to someone who is not drinking ACV daily.

Eat potassium

Potassium is the miracle ingredient of health. Eat fruits and vegetables high in potassium. It reduces stress levels and lowers blood pressure. High stress levels are known to prompt our body to store fat, and put on weight.

Additionally, potassium is an electrolyte; it is responsible for the flow of electromagnetic energy in the body.

Also, our body is not very good at retaining potassium. It is therefore very important to eat lots of fresh fruits and vegetables. Ideally aim to have three servings of vegetables and two servings of fruits every day. One serving is roughly the size of your fist.

Lower sugar intake

While fruits contain sugar, if you eat them within limit, this tip will not contradict with the previous tip. Make sure you are eating less refined sugar. Refined or processed sugar adds unwanted calories to our diet, makes us lethargic, drains out energy and creates craving for more. Don't remove sugar completely and suddenly, lest it should cause withdrawal symptoms. Gradually reduce the sugar content so that your palette gets used to low sugar diet.

I have reduced the amount of sugar I put in my tea from 3 teaspoons to 1 teaspoon gradually. Our taste buds are clever; they soon re-adjust to the new taste by increasing their sensitivity. Not only does my tea taste as good, the new habit has had a spillover effect on other foods. I have developed an aversion to sugar-heavy desserts. Because my body is not trying hard to process too much sugar, I feel more energetic.

Laugh out loud

Laughter is the best medicine, they say. And rightly so.

Laughing helps to exercise stomach muscles. It improves our breathing, increases supply of blood around the body, which in turn causes body to burn fat. Laughter also reduces stress, and produces serotonin – the 'feel good' chemical in our body. Feeling good about ourselves gives us renewed confidence to stay on the path of healthy life.

So grab your favorite DVD of a funny movie or TV series, and laugh your guts out.

Avoid hard liquor

Alcohol contains calories that you can do without. Alcohol is also mixed with other drinks that are high in caffeine or sugar. All these factors are counter-productive to your weight loss goals. However, there is a bigger problem caused by alcohol. It is known to interfere with muscle building. It also reduces our blood's ability to carry oxygen around. All this makes it difficult to reach your weight-loss goals.

Still not convinced? Alcohol also reduces the quality of sleep we experience. Poor sleeping patterns deprive us of much-needed rest, increases stress levels and leads to craving for more food. I am not suggesting that you should become a teetotaler. Drink in moderation. Better still, drink red wine. It is full of anti-oxidants and has good anti-aging effect. Did you realize that red wine is related to vinegar?

Apple cider vinegar energizes from within, and gives a natural high. As cider vinegar becomes a habit, you will be less inclined to pursue alcohol.

Take vitamins and minerals supplements

Body needs lots of vitamins and minerals to work optimally. They are essential for maintenance of body cells, developing strength, building immunity and leading an active life. Millions of years ago, when man lived in the Savannah forest, he received ample supply of these essential foods from fruits and vegetables growing in the natural environment.

In the modern age, commercially produced fruits and vegetables lack sufficient supply of nutrients. Modern lifestyle has also reduced our intake of healthy food and increased the consumption of diet high in sodium and fat. This is why vitamins and minerals supplements are a must, even if you are eating plenty of green stuff.

Taking supplements is even more important if you are exercising regularly. Physical exercise, whether it is running, swimming or weight-lifting, produces free radicals. Also, the air we breathe contains free radicals. An athlete breathes more air than a sedentary person, and is more exposed to free radicals. Lastly, physically active person loses a lot of vitamins and minerals through sweat and urination. Consult your doctor for a good brand of multi-vitamins and minerals supplements.

11. BETTER HAIR WITH ACV

Apple cider vinegar is popularly used to improve the health of hair: get shiny hair, boost hair growth, and remove dandruff. ACV can replace expensive hair-care treatment., since the regular use of ACV can strengthen hair by restoring its protective layer, while also keeping the scalp clean. The potassium in apple cider vinegar is tonic for our hair, feeding it with the much-needed mineral. Similarly, malic acid in ACV helps to cure fungal and bacterial infections. Apple cider vinegar works in many ways to improve the quality of hair.

Cleansing

ACV rinse is good for removing nasty chemicals and pollutants from the hair. It can even be mixed with baking soda for better cleansing. In fact, a mix of ACV and baking soda acts as both shampoo as well as conditioner. I'll discuss the best use ACV and baking soda later in this chapter.

pH balancing factor

Many expensive shampoos and conditioners are advertised for their pH balancing benefit. ACV does this job naturally and for a lot less money. Why would you then flush your money down the drain? Washing hair with regular shampoo increases the pH factor of our hair. (pH factor is an indicator of acidity level. Anything between 0 and 6 is acidic.) In its natural form, our hair are acidic, with a pH factor of 4 to 6. Apple cider vinegar has a pH factor of about 4. Thus, washing hair with ACV restores the pH balance after shampooing hair.

Shiny, Smooth Hair

Because ACV rinse helps in smoothing the hair, it reduces split hair. When combined with baking soda, ACV gives a nice, shiny look to the hair.

Dandruff

As ACV clears up dead cells (dandruff) built up on scalp, you will experience less itchiness. ACV's antibacterial and anti-fungal properties help in removing infection from hair, and stops scratchiness. Additionally, apple cider vinegar is known to treat Alopecia. It is also used to treat hair (scalp) psoriasis, as I'll discuss later in the book.

Making Apple Cider Vinegar Hair Rinse

Take one part of organic apple cider vinegar and mix it with one part warm water. Use distilled water preferably.

Also, it is advisable to use lukewarm water. Hot water weakens hair and makes it fragile. Cold water may not be able to remove dandruff and may prevent ACV from reaching to the scalp.

There are some variations of ACV rinse which you may want to try. You can add baking soda to apple cider vinegar rinse, to get shiny and healthy hair. You may even add aloe vera to it.

Washing Hair with ACV rinse

My preference is to avoid shampoo completely. Simply wash your hair with ACV rinse. No need for shampoo or conditioner. However, many people struggle to get over the habit of using a shampoo.

In which case, use ACV rinse in place of a conditioner. Wash your hair normally with your favorite shampoo. Get rid of excess water with a gentle towel dry. While your hair is still wet, rub the apple cider vinegar rinse in to your hair and scalp.

Unlike a regular conditioner, ACV should get massaged into the scalp. This will help in removing harmful chemicals and dandruff from the hair. Let ACV get absorbed in the scalp for 15 minutes. Rinse hair as usual.

Choosing The Right ACV For Hair Rinse

Many commercial ACV products are not good for hair. Buy raw unheated, unpasteurized, unfiltered ACV. Such unpasteurized cider vinegar contains the "mother" of

ACV, which provides the essential enzymes. Buy organic preferably.

For hair, you can either use liquid ACV or powder ACV. I have used liquid ACV and found it very beneficial in treating my hair. I prefer to use it undiluted because the hair is already wet when ACV is applied. First-time users should dilute it initially until they are sure that their scalp is not sensitive to ACV.

ACV Takes Time

I am often asked - how long does it take for ACV to stop hair fall if I am using ACV regularly?

Apple cider vinegar is not a quick fix for hair loss. You will need to give it some time. In my case, I have used it for over a year. Now it has become a second nature. It is not just the hair growth benefits that I use it for. I use ACV for improving the health of my hair.

I don't need any shampoo or conditioner now. I also mix ACV rinse with baking soda once a month. This gives a nice shine to my hair. Remember, baking soda is harsh. I wouldn't recommend using baking soda more than once a month to wash hair. ACV can be used for lifetime. Even after you notice the benefits of ACV use, continue to use it to keep hair in good health. I use it for its antibacterial and anti-fungal benefits.

As you keep using it regularly, you will get used to the smell, which is a put-off initially. Because I was already drinking ACV regularly, I was used to the smell. If you are concerned about the smell, you can use ACV rinse less frequently.

Each person may report unique results. The results may depend on the person's natural disposition, the quality of water, and the environment. To get the most benefits for hair growth, application of ACV should be supplemented by taking ACV internally. Drink ACV regularly as described earlier in this book so as to provide internal nourishment to hair.

As with other things, cider vinegar alone cannot help in stopping hair fall. Hair loss occurs because of a combination of reasons - stress, smoking, unhealthy food, pollution, shampoo, ultra-violet rays, hard water, just to name a few.

To be able to stop hair loss, you must make lifestyle changes. Eat healthy. Exercise regularly. Use distilled water to wash hair. Sleep well. Take vitamins and minerals supplements regularly as per doctor's prescription.

Even if your hair loss is caused by genetic factors, you can arrest hair fall and may even be able to reverse it, by following healthy lifestyle described in this book.

12. ACV FOR GLOWING SKIN

Skincare is one of the most important benefits of apple cider vinegar. It is used for treating acne, warts, zits, and for getting youthful skin. ACV makes skin look younger and feel smoother. Before I get into the method of using apple cider vinegar for skincare, let me spend a moment to explain why looking after skin is absolutely essential for overall health.

Researchers have found that two of the biggest factors that influence the attractiveness of a person are skin and hair. Skin is the largest organ of our body. It accounts for 16 percent of our weight and is 2 square meters in area. It comprises two layers – the outer epidermis and the inner dermis.

A key role played by skin is providing protection at the surface of the body. But there's one more role that skin plays which is equally important- receiving sensory stimuli. As the largest medium for receiving feedback from our surroundings – the skin acts as the touch and feel tool of communication.

In fact, touch is one of the most important forms of bonding not just in humans, but in animals and birds too. From the tuck of a mother, to buddy-punching, a romantic kiss and an empathetic hug, touch is to the core of social relationships, and such bonding is only possible with healthy skin.

In fact, quality of skin is considered to be a good indicator of the quality of health of a person. Pale skin is a sign of unhealthy body. Glowing and youthful skin exhibits health.

And if you don't have good skin, don't worry. Our body is regularly making new skin that replaces existing skin. Even as you are reading this, your body is quietly making a new layer under your skin. And it doesn't take us long to make new skin. We have completely new skin every 30 days or so.

Healthy skin helps to maintain a healthy body. It does so by performing important bodily functions:

- Receiving and conveying information to external stimuli
- Controlling body temperature
- Protecting from ultra-violet rays, physical dangers, harmful bacteria and other undesirable elements of the environment

Apple cider vinegar is our friend in our endeavor to

getting healthy skin.

ACV Cure For Acne, Pimples

Apple cider vinegar is very effective for skincare, for treating acne and pimples. It can even be mixed in honey and applied on an open wound to stop bleeding. Both honey and apple cider vinegar have anti-bacterial properties. You could keep a small bottle of cider vinegar in your car and use it to stop bleeding as well as to treat burn injury.

Our skin's renewal function (replacing old cells with new cells) is hindered when the top layer of dead cells remains on skin, prohibiting the new skin from taking over. ACV is effective in removing these dead cells, as well as unblocking pores so that our skin can breathe properly. Additionally, it helps in creating a protective layer on skin, and preventing skin from becoming too dry.

How Does ACV Work For Skin

To stay healthy, our skin needs to remain well-hydrated. However modern day living and working conditions often make our skin dry.

Skin has a protective layer called *protective acid mantle*. As the name suggests, it is this acidity that offers protection to our skin. Its acidic nature guards us from pollution, free radicals and other harmful particles in the air. Our acidic skin in its natural form has a pH factor of 4.5 to 6. Constant exposure to the sunlight makes skin dry. Even the water we use to wash face contains chlorine that damages the protective layer. Our regular face-wash also removes the protective acid mantle.

If it weren't exposed to the sun, water and face-wash, our skin would mostly remain healthy and keep us healthy. It would do so by naturally replenishing the damaged protective acid mantle. This process takes time, and in modern living conditions, we are removing the protective layer faster than our body has time to heal and replenish it.

In the absence of this acidic protection, skin remains exposed to harmful elements around us. Such prolonged exposure causes skin diseases including rashes, pimples and acne.

Don't Despair, ACV Is Here

Apple cider vinegar has a three-pronged approach in restoring the health of our skin.

1. At the basic level, apple cider vinegar acts as an antiseptic and antibacterial cream, which offers cure from bacterial and viral infection.

2. Beta-carotene in ACV is one of the most important elements for our health. It protects us from cancer. Beta-carotene is effective in fighting free radicals.

3. The most obvious and direct benefit of apple cider vinegar is its ability to restore the pH balance of the skin. Apple cider vinegar has a pH factor of about 4.5 to 5.5, which is very close to the ideal pH factor for human skin too. Of course, you should not use ACV straight from

the bottle. You need to make an ACV toner for use on skin.

Making ACV Toner

You can easily make apple cider vinegar toner for skin at home. What you need:

- 200 ml distilled water (tap water is also fine, if you have no choice).
- 200 ml apple cider vinegar, only unfiltered and unpasteurized (so that it contains the 'mother' of vinegar)
- 500 ml plastic bottle, to store apple cider vinegar toner

Method

Fill a sterilized 500 ml bottle with 200 ml filtered water in it. Now fill it up with apple cider vinegar of equal quantity. You are mixing one part water with one part ACV.

Shake the bottle well. Your apple cider vinegar toner is ready. Before each use, make sure you shake the bottle so that the mother of vinegar gets mixed.

Using ACV toner for better skin

Put some toner on a cotton pad or ball and gently wipe it on your skin. Avoid contact with eyes.

Begin gradually by using it once a day and then increase the frequency to twice a day. This will allow you to test the sensitivity of your skin.

For the same reason, try ACV on a small area of your skin first. If skin gets irritable, add more water to the toner.

Apply ACV toner preferably at night because the smell of ACV could be too strong for a social set up.

When using for the first time, you should wash it off after 5 minutes so that your skin is not exposed to ACV for too long initially. You want to introduce ACV to your skin gradually. Once you are comfortable with it, you may leave it on overnight. For the difficult-to-reach areas like back, put it in a spray bottle and use. Let the skin absorb it.

While I have recommended a 1:1 ratio for mixing ACV with water – you may want to experiment with it. Each person's skin is unique, as is his or her DNA. If irritation occurs, add more water. If you are comfortable, you may reduce the quantity of water.

Some people mix 2 part ACV with one part water. However always start with a 1:1 or higher ratio of water, and then decrease the water quantity to arrive at the best ratio for your skin.

Similarly, don't apply undiluted apple cider vinegar on skin. ACV is acidic, and can damage skin if exposed to undiluted ACV for too long. However, I have feedback from readers who have reported amazing results by applying undiluted cider vinegar on skin. But I would advise caution initially.

Also, avoid using cider vinegar in areas around the eyes. If ACV enters your eyes, wash it off with clean water. If irritation persists, see your doctor.

You could add half a cup cider vinegar to your bath water and soak yourself in it for about 15 to 30 minutes. This will help in removing dead cells, as well as opening the pores on the skin.

Many people experiment with other beneficial ingredients such as green tea, aloe vera gel, or witch hazel to ACV to get more health benefits from your toner.

Choosing the Right Apple Cider Vinegar

The normal filtered, distilled white vinegar is not suitable for making apple cider vinegar toner. Apple cider vinegar needs to be unpasteurized and unfiltered. I prefer organic apple cider vinegar, especially for applying on face since it is not harsh on skin.

I prefer to use ACV toner at night - soon after dinner. I wash my face with face-wash and apply ACV toner, however this is not essential. You could simply dampen your face with warm water and gently dry it with a towel, before applying ACV toner. I feel fresh immediately, though the smell puts off my partner. So I wash it off before getting into bed.

I have found apple cider vinegar effective in preventing acne, though it takes a long time to remove existing acne. It is not an overnight remedy. I use it for the cleansing benefit. ACV is effective for treating blackheads too. ACV opens the pores and makes it easier to clean blackheads.

Precautions before using ACV on skin

Apple cider vinegar toner is very useful for treating skin diseases like acne, pimples and other ailments. However, read these tips before using apple cider vinegar for skincare.

- Some people may find the smell too strong. Actually, apple cider vinegar smells like sweaty socks that you forgot under the bed for two weeks. Just as you wouldn't eat raw onion or garlic before a date, you wouldn't wear apple cider vinegar on face if you were stepping out. If you can't stand the smell, simply use it at night.

- While apple cider vinegar is usually incident-free toner to use, in some cases, it may cause skin irritation. Some people may have extra sensitive skin, and apple cider vinegar may not be suitable for them. However, before giving up completely on apple cider vinegar, try to further dilute it with water, and you may find that the irritation subsides after a while. Alternatively, reduce the frequency of using apple cider vinegar.

- In very rare situations, some people may experience purging. If purging happens you may want to stop using apple cider vinegar. Purging happens when ACV opens up blockages on skin and your skin pushes out impurities. So your existing pimples may get redder and get worse before getting better.

- At first, use ACV on a small part of skin, and see how it reacts. Use generously diluted ACV first and get feedback.

- Use of apple cider vinegar toner on skin can increase

13. DIABETES CURE WITH ACV

Apple cider vinegar is known to be useful for people with diabetes.

In a study entitled *"Therapeutic Effect Of Daily Vinegar Ingestion For Individuals At Risk For Type 2 Diabetes"*[9] conducted by Carol S. Johnston, Samantha Quagliano, and Serena Whit from School of Nutrition and Health Promotion, Arizona State University, organic unpasteurized apple cider vinegar was given to a test group over a period of 12 weeks. They drank ACV before meal in the morning. The data from the study indicate "daily vinegar consumption favorably influences fasting glucose concentrations in healthy adults, and contribute important information to the growing evidence base supporting the antiglycemic effects of vinegar".

"Vinegar ingestion at mealtime reduces postprandial glycemia and increases satiety, metabolic effects that may benefit individuals struggling with diabetes."

The study supported health benefits of consuming ACV not just as a drink but also as part of cooking. "Vinegar can be incorporated into meals as a vinaigrette dressing on salads or vegetables or as a sandwich spread in the form of mustard, or it can simply be spritzed onto foods."

The study also recommended using apple cider vinegar drink instead of ACV pills so as to get health benefits. "Commercial vinegar tablets do not contain adequate amounts of acetic acid to induce an antiglycemic effect," the researchers found.

Another view is that cider vinegar slows down digestion, which in turn causes glucose to be released slowly in the blood. This helps in avoiding the typical post-prandial (post-meal) drastic rise in glucose level, which is a major problem faced by diabetics. Cider vinegar ensures that glucose enters the system in a moderate fashion, giving time to pancreas to match up the glucose with insulin.

Diabetic patients already on medication for diabetes must consult their doctor, since consumption of ACV may have an additive effect and cause blood sugar levels to drop to an undesirable level.

14. TREATING UTI

Urinary tract infection is a common infection which is very painful and embarrassing. If ignored, UTI can cause serious medical complications, and should not be ignored.

Urinary Tract Infection Symptoms

Common as it is, UTI can be unbearable. It begins as a burning sensation, and develops into stomach pain, backache and fever.

Many women dismiss it as period pain in the beginning. Here are the main symptoms of urinary tract infection:

- Burning sensation
- Strong urge to visit washroom often
- Dark and cloudy urine with foul smell
- Fever and chill

Women get UTI more often than men, though it is not rare for men to be infected.

Women's anatomy makes them more vulnerable to urinary tract infection - women have shorter urinary tract. Besides, vagina and anus is located very close to each other. This makes it easier for bacteria to enter urinary tract via vagina.

Urinary Tract Infection Causes

UTI is caused when bacteria enters urinary tract and our body is unable to fight the infection. Let's look at the anatomy to understand causes of UTI. This will also help in understanding various types of UTI.

When we eat food it is processed in such a way that nutrients are absorbed in the blood and waste products are removed from the body. Our liquid waste, which is urine, is gathered in the bladder, where it stays until removed from body. When we visit washroom, this urine passes from bladder to urethra which is a thin pipe which takes the urine out of the body.

This is a one-way street, but sometimes UTI-causing bacteria manage to enter urethra, and cause **urethritis** - infection of the urethra. Sometimes the bacteria may not be satisfied with infecting urethra, and may move up the tract into bladder. The infection of bladder is called **cystitis**.

Remember, our body contains trillions of bacteria. In fact our gut and our digestion system is home to many different types of bacteria. Some of these are good bacteria, which are essential for good digestion. We get these bacteria from food, especially yogurt.

However, our body is host to bad bacteria too. Our immune system takes care of them, and we don't even notice an infection. Every infection doesn't result in a disease and can remain asymptomatic as long as our immune system has successfully managed it.

When the body's army fails to fight the infection, we fall sick. Most of the times, the UTI infection is kept under control by our immune system. But stubborn bacteria win in some cases.

The main causes of UTI are:

- Inadequate hygiene in toilets
- Poor vaginal cleanliness
- Sexual intercourse
- Weak immune system

How To Treat UTI With Vinegar

Two most popular remedies for UTI are apple cider vinegar and cranberries. Cider vinegar is not only effective in treating UTI but also in preventing it. Potassium, enzymes and minerals in cider vinegar are effective in fighting disease-causing bacteria. Cider vinegar also has an antibiotic effect, as mentioned earlier in this book. However, in case of severe infection, it is best to consult a doctor, because UTI could cause serious damage to organs if it is not controlled with medical treatment. Apple cider vinegar has the best chance of fighting infection if it is consumed as soon as first signs of UTI are observed. It is also effective in preventing UTI if it is made part of everyday diet.

How To Drink Cider Vinegar

Take a cup of warm water, preferably distilled, and put a couple of teaspoons of cider vinegar in it. Drink this two to three times a day, ideally on an empty stomach. You could also add organic honey or maple syrup to it, which is optional.

If you are susceptible to recurring UTI, you may wish to drink ACV regularly. Make one liter of ACV drink in the morning, and carry the bottle with you to work or college. Drinking ACV regularly will not only strengthen immunity but also provide a strong energy boost.

Give ACV three to five days to be effective, though many people report improvement within 24 hours. However, if the pain is severe, or in case of an acute episode of UTI, consult your doctor immediately; urinary tract infection may cause serious damage to internal organs if it is not treated in time.

The Right Vinegar for UTI

As with other sections of this book, this section would also recommend unfiltered, unpasteurized cider vinegar. Ordinary white vinegar will not do the trick. Preferably buy organic cider vinegar.

Other Home Remedies for UTI

Cranberry Juice

Cranberry juice is full of proanthocyanidins, which prohibits E.Coli and other bacteria from sticking to the walls of urinary tract. This helps in easy removal of the bacteria from the body. Drink 100% cranberry juice daily.

Baking Soda

Baking soda is commonly used to treat UTI. It influences the pH level of urine, and gives quick relief from the unbearable pain caused by UTI. Put one teaspoon of soda in a cup of water and drink it once a day.

Tea Tree Oil

Add one teaspoon of tea tree oil a bottle of water and wipe vaginal area with the mixture. Tea tree oil is effective in killing bacteria.

Antibiotics and UTI

Because UTI could lead to more critical health issues, it is important to visit a doctor and get on an antibiotics course if UTI shows no sign of improvement. However, UTI could be a recurring infection, and antibiotics may fail to be effective if bacteria develop resistance over a period of time.

This is why it is important to keep UTI at bay, by using natural products like cider vinegar, cranberries and vitamin

C supplements. These home remedies offer a long-term solution in fighting UTI while antibiotics should be considered as an immediate and short-term defense.

When ACV May Not Be Effective

As we have discussed, UTI is bacterial infection. To cure UTI, we have two options - either kill the bacteria, or remove it from the body. Apple cider vinegar can help in removing bacteria in most cases, including E.Coli, which are the most common UTI-causing bacteria.

Cider vinegar is also effective in preventing the growth of bacteria. However, certain bacteria are very stubborn and may not respond to natural treatment like cider vinegar. These are typically gram-positive bacteria like staph saprophyticus. Staph usually causes UTI of bladder in young women. Staph is difficult to be washed out of the body with cider vinegar. You will need to actively kill it with medication.

UTI treatment therefore will depend on the bacteria. This is why it is important to know which bacteria are causing urinary infection. If you are experiencing a recurring infection, chances are it is caused by the same bacteria. You will need to choose your treatment according to the bacteria. Cider vinegar can help in washing out some bacteria, as well as preventing the growth of bad bacteria in urinary tract.

Other effective treatments for E.Coli are D-Mannose tablets, cranberry juice or Cystex tablets.

Prevent Urinary Tract Infection

- Drink sufficient water. Our body is 70% water, and drinking distilled water not only strengthens immunity but also helps in flushing out bacteria.

- Drink organic cider vinegar every day.

- Avoid aerated/carbonated drinks.

- Introduce yogurt in your breakfast or lunch.

- Don't be frugal with your visits to washroom; go as often as you can.

- Women should urinate before and after sexual intercourse, and then drink a glass of water.

- Avoid anal and vaginal intercourse consequently.

- After urination, women should wipe vaginal area with a tissue - front to back. Move the tissue from vagina to anus, and not the other way.

- For women suffering from a gram-positive bacteria, drinking baking soda water regularly could help in maintaining the pH factor of your urine high, which stops the growth of bacteria.

- Here's the most important tip - take vitamin C tablets or cranberry tablets every day so as to build immunity.

15. TREATING PSORIASIS

Psoriasis is a non-contagious skin disease. When immune system mistakenly considers the cells in skin as pathogens (an infectious agent), it begins to attack those cells by producing more cells to fight.

If not treated in time, psoriasis can cause more serious health conditions. According to *American Academy of Dermatology*,[10] people in their 40s with severe psoriasis were more than twice as likely to suffer a heart attack than people without the skin disease. These findings were based on medical records of more than 680,000 British patients.

Types of psoriasis of the skin

Chronic plaque psoriasis: This is the most common psoriasis that causes either silver or white colored patches called plaques. While plaques usually develop on knees and elbows, they can spread all over the body including private body parts. These plaques could be small or large.

Hair psoriasis or psoriasis of the scalp: When psoriasis develops on the scalp, it is known as hair psoriasis. People suffering from plaque psoriasis are likely to develop scalp psoriasis at some stage. Which is why a dermatologist needs to take a scalp sample to confirm hair psoriasis and recommend treatment. Usual remedies for treating psoriasis on other parts of the body are not suitable for scalp, which is much thicker skin.

Psoriatic arthritis: These patches develop at the joints and result in inflammation.

What causes psoriasis

Existing research hasn't conclusively explained causes of psoriasis, though we know it is an autoimmune disease which rarely gets cured and lasts for a lifetime. The only exception is psoriasis of the scalp, which is treatable. It is widely believed to have been caused by stress, smoking, alcohol or trauma to the skin.

Psoriasis cures

Unfortunately, no known cures exist that are effective in eradicating psoriasis completely, though many remedies are used to manage the outbreak.

How apple cider vinegar cures psoriasis

Very little clinical evidence exists to support the effectiveness of cider vinegar for treating psoriasis. However, many people around the world have shared their positive experiences of treating psoriasis with cider vinegar. It is not clear how apple cider vinegar works to cure psoriasis; one explanation is the cider vinegar's ability to balance the pH factor. Our diet and usually our living conditions disturb the pH balance of our bodies as well as that of skin. Apple cider vinegar helps in re-balancing our pH factor. ACV helps by breaking down the plaques, and when used with a steroid cream, allows the medicine to absorb better to heal and prevent psoriasis more effectively.

How to apply cider vinegar

There are two ways of using apple cider vinegar for skin diseases, including psoriasis:

* Externally - by applying directly on skin
* Internally - by drinking diluted cider vinegar

Applying cider vinegar on skin

Apple cider vinegar is acidic, and helps in restoring pH balance of the skin. It is also antibacterial, and assists in fighting free radicals from the skin. Take a cup and fill it up half with water and half with cider vinegar. Mix ACV and water in 1:1 ratio. Use a piece of cloth, cotton ball, or cotton pad, and dab it in the diluted ACV and apply it on the affected area. Leave it for about half an hour and rinse it off. I have received feedback from people who prefer to apply cider vinegar on skin without diluting it. While this could be effective, begin with diluted cider vinegar, and once you are sure that your skin can handle it, try undiluted cider vinegar. Apply it twice a day for best results.

Topically apply cider to pimples, acne and warts too. Caution: always try it out on a small part of skin, preferably hidden skin, in case skin should break out.

Drinking apple cider vinegar

Apple cider vinegar is effective in treating psoriasis when used not just externally but also internally. Consumption of apple cider vinegar offers a range of benefits. Drink apple cider vinegar twice a day, preferably on an empty stomach. Never drink cider vinegar without diluting it first. It has 5% acidity and may cause damage to teeth enamel. Take a cup of water, put two to three teaspoons of cider vinegar and drink it. Add honey to it to improve its taste. I prefer organic honey usually.

Other treatments for psoriasis

Here are some of the common cures used by people suffering from psoriasis. You may want to see what works.

- Banana leaves
- Aloe vera
- Coconut oil, castor oil
- Baking soda
- Beet juice
- Turmeric
- Shea butter
- Hydrogen peroxide
- Glycerin

16. TREATING VARICOSE VEINS

"I have suffered for months now with extreme swelling of my legs. After (consulting) many specialists, I took matters in my own hands. Unprocessed apple cider vinegar has not only eased the edema, my varicose veins have almost totally disappeared! If I didn't see with my own eyes I would never have imagined. I drink two teaspoons in water twice a day. The best!"

Tucker from Virginia Beach, Va, the United States (Source: *The Earth Clinic*[11]**)**

Varicose veins or spider veins are usually red or blue veins that appear on the surface of legs. Blood vessels or veins in body, especially legs, have valves to regulate the flow of blood so that blood traveling up from legs towards heart doesn't flow backwards. These valves effectively ensure that blood flows one way - upwards.

In case of people with varicose veins, these valves are either partially or fully damaged, or are missing. As a result, blood flows backwards and accumulates in the veins, causing swelling. Obviously, this swelling is usually more prominent when you are standing or sitting for too long.

How to use apple cider vinegar

Take cheesecloth or medical cloth used for bandage. Soak it in apple cider vinegar, and tie it around thighs or lower legs. Leave it on for half an hour. Remove the bandage, and wash your legs. Because apple cider vinegar is acidic, you may first want to experiment with a very small area of your skin. Sensitive skin may develop rash with the use of apple cider vinegar.

For better results, lie down on flat surface and put a few pillows under ankles, so that blood flow is reduced to legs. Another way to use apple cider vinegar is to apply it directly on legs. Word of caution: this may cause a rash; try it on a small part of a leg to see whether your skin is sensitive to cider vinegar. Supplement this external application with internal consumption. Drink apple cider vinegar twice a day. Put two to three teaspoon of apple cider vinegar, in a cup of water and drink before meals. For better taste, add one teaspoon of organic honey to the ACV drink. This should help in removing the inflammation of veins. Results may vary, and may take about a month for any visible signs of improvement.

Other natural remedies for varicose veins

Spider veins can leave your legs looking ugly, if the veins look red or blue. Use these natural solutions to treat varicose veins:

- Eat one garlic clove a day - raw. Peel a garlic clove, crush it by hand, and then swallow it down with water - like a pill.

- Mix one-teaspoon of cayenne pepper in a cup of warm water and drink it twice or thrice a day. This helps in relieving the pain in the legs. It improves the blood flow. This may take 15 to 20 days to cure varicose veins. After that, drink it once a day to stay healthy.

- Cod liver oil can be mixed with honey and applied to a bandage. Tie this bandage and leave it overnight. It helps in removing the swelling.

Preventing varicose veins

With some precautions, it is possible to prevent varicose veins. Exercise regularly. Exercise improves blood flow and helps in better weight management, which in turn may help in lowering chances of varicose veins. Light exercise like walking is good for preventing varicose veins. Also massaging your legs regularly also helps in improving blood circulation and preventing varicose veins. However, not all exercise is good. In fact, strenuous exercise may worsen existing varicose veins, as it may put too much pressure on the valves. Avoid long-distance running, or heavy weight-lifting, unless it is recommended by a doctor. However, light exercises like walking, flexing ankle muscles, simple calf-raises could help in preventing as well reducing varicose veins (Source: *WebMD*[12]).

Some more ways to prevent blue veins:

- Manage weight. Putting too much pressure of weight on legs decreases our ability to be mobile.

- Don't spend too much time in a sitting or standing position. Take a walk every now and then, even if it means just walking to the printer in the office, or popping out in the backyard.

- Avoid high heel footwear.

- Use sunscreen while out. Exposure to strong sun can also cause blue veins on the face.

- Diet: reduce salt content. Modern diet contains too much salt. Eat lots of veggies, and a handful of fruits. Eat lentils, and any food high in fiber and low in sodium.

- Drink plenty of water so that your bowel movements are regular. Constipation can worsen blue veins.

- Wear compressive stockings.

If your condition has reached an extreme state and all natural remedies fail, you may want to consider surgical intervention: saphenous vein stripping.

Varicose Vein Stripping

In extreme cases, natural remedies may not work, and the only option left will be going under the knife. Your doctor will be able to advise the best solution for advanced varicose veins. In most cases, doctors recommend varicose vein stripping.

This is a surgical procedure performed to cure varicose veins. In this surgery, the damaged vein is either tied off or removed completely. This surgery is performed either with general anesthesia or spinal anesthesia.

Since the surgery involves removal of a vein, it is the last option to consider while treating spider veins. It should not be treated as a cosmetic surgery and should be opted for only if you experience excruciating pain in legs, or if there are blood clots or swelling.

17. OTHER HEALTH USES OF ACV

Apples are loaded with minerals, primarily potassium, which help in delaying age-related deterioration of health. Potassium is an important mineral for rejuvenating tired tissues in our body. It helps in repairing soft tissues.

Lack of potassium causes hair loss. It also makes our teeth weak. Apple cider vinegar is full of potassium, and helps in fighting issues related to bones, teeth and hair fall. It also contains calcium, which maintains the health of bones and prevents them from becoming fragile with age.

ACV helps in fixing the acid-alkaline balance (pH factor) of the body, protecting us from common cold, and speeding up recovery from minor illnesses. It contains plenty of antioxidants that help prevent cancer and are effective anti-ageing agents. Apple cider vinegar is a must-have food in every kitchen because of its many applications and uses in daily life.

Cider Vinegar - The Nectar of Life

Apple cider vinegar offers a range of health benefits:

- Improves digestion
- Boosts immune system
- Promotes healthy skin
- Restores pH balance in hair and skin
- Removes toxins from body
- Reduces joint pain and muscle ache

For centuries, human race has been using apple cider for better health and skin. Made from organic apples, cider vinegar can be stored at room temperature and has a long shelf life. It doesn't need refrigeration.

Cider vinegar is used in our daily activities, right from drinking it for weight loss, applying it on hair as a conditioner, rubbing it on skin for glowing skin, and to use it for other health benefits. Let's find out the many uses of apple cider vinegar in daily life.

Dental Cleaning

Apple cider vinegar for clean teeth? Yes, ACV can be used for dental hygiene. It can help in killing oral bacteria, remove tartar (plaque), protect from gum disease, whiten teeth and prevent bad breath. But before you get excited, read this carefully. To clean teeth with ACV, take one or two teaspoon of cider vinegar and mix it with one cup of lukewarm water. After brushing teeth, rinse mouth with this ACV water. Rinse it a couple of times. Then rinse mouth with clean water. This is important. Cider vinegar is acidic and may damage teeth.

Some people even follow the ACV rinse with baking soda rinse. Simply mix a spoon of baking soda in half a cup of water and rinse mouth with baking soda, after you have rinsed with ACV water. Baking soda removes ACV from the mouth and also helps in whitening teeth. Follow the baking soda rinse by clean water rinse. You don't want baking soda to stay on your teeth either.

Because of its acidic quality, ACV helps in killing bacteria built up in mouth. Isn't that a very effective way to fight bad breath?

Foot spa

Apple cider vinegar can be used in pedicure, to soothe tired feet. Add half a cup of apple cider vinegar to foot spa water, and gently soak your feet in. You will feel the muscles in your feet relax as the skin soaks in the vinegar.

Because of its acidic nature, cider vinegar also kills bacteria and germs from feet, leaving the skin refreshingly smooth and odorless. A word of caution: don't leave your skin in ACV water for too long. Moderate foot bath for about half an hour is advisable.

This provides relief for tired feet for people who do a lot of walking, and for pregnant women, runners and anyone who has to stand for long duration in their job.

For people with heel pain (sometimes referred to as calcaneal spur or heel spur), cider vinegar can help relieve the constant ache. Cut a piece of paper in the the shape of foot, soak this paper in cider vinegar and place foot on it. Keep it for about 15 minutes, and discard the paper. Alternatively, dab a cotton ball in cider vinegar, and gently wipe foot, allowing cider vinegar to be soaked in. This will help relax foot muscles.

Deodorant

While apple cider vinegar has a strong smell, it acts as a good deodorant. Apply it in diluted form to underarms and other sweaty areas of the body; it kills strong body odors. ACV even helps in keeping our skin healthy because of its anti-bacterial properties. Dilute ACV in water and fill up a spray bottle. Spray after shower, and walk out confidently. For the first few minutes, the odor of ACV will dominate; this will subside. Make sure to use it in diluted form, as it may sting in sensitive areas or on cut skin.

Sunburn

For people from regions with heavy UV-ray exposure, apple cider vinegar can be applied on the sun-burnt skin. Soak a piece of cloth or cotton ball in ACV water and apply on the affected area. It will soothe the burning sensation and help the skin recover sooner.

Remember, if your skin is sensitive to apple cider vinegar, avoid using ACV for sunburn injury.

Bath

Add a few spoons of organic apple cider vinegar to your bathtub, and let the skin soak in the vinegar. This will not only have anti-bacterial benefit, but also help in relaxing tense muscles. Did I mention glowing skin as a by-product of apple cider vinegar bath?

Digestion

Most of us suffer from stomach issues every now and then. If you have diarrhea, put one to three teaspoon cider vinegar and one-teaspoon honey in one glass of lukewarm water and drink it. ACV helps in forming fibrous matter, which cures diarrhea. Similarly, people suffering from regular episodes of indigestion will find relief in apple cider vinegar. Put one spoon of ACV in water and drink it an hour before meal. This will prevent a stomach upset or that bloated feeling. Apple cider vinegar assists the digestive juices in the gut, promotes the growth of 'gut flora' (good bacteria), and helps in removing waste products from stomach. As a result, digestion improves and so does energy level as explained next.

Energy

These days, we lead hectic lifestyle, which further gets compounded by a lack of physical activity and exercise. Fatigue follows because of the lactic acid produced by the body. Enzymes in apple cider vinegar act as a balancing factor. Potassium in ACV gives us that energy boost. Add a spoon of ACV to water and drink. Take it as a sport drink during your run or gym workout.

18. ACV FOR PETS

Cider vinegar is a great source of minerals for most animals. My guinea pigs get a regular feed of cider vinegar - mixed in their drip-water-bottle. Initially they did not like the taste of vinegar; so I gradually introduced it to them. Now they are more energetic and have shiny fur - which is a good indication of their health. Not only guinea pigs but also other animals benefit from cider vinegar.

You can feed organic cider vinegar to:

* Chickens
* Sheep
* Dogs
* Cats
* Horses
* Other pets

Here's a story about feeding cider vinegar to chicken. Paul Bragg, the man who devoted his life to cider vinegar and built a successful business around it (remember Bragg Apple Cider Vinegar?), shares this story in his book, "*Apple Cider Vinegar Miracle Health System*".[13] Paul describes how the children in the Bragg family were introduced to the benefits of cider vinegar. The grandfather once selected an old hen for dinner. The children noticed that the old hen's meat was "tough and didn't taste good".

He then selected another old hen, and gave her cider vinegar twice a day, for ten days. When this hen was served for dinner, the meat was tender, "just like a young hen".

It can be added to the water of chickens, horses and sheep. The beneficial value of vinegar lies in the minerals in it. Vinegar also regulates metabolism and blood sugar, which may explain the usefulness of vinegar to animals.

Benefits of cider vinegar for pets:

- Keeps away parasites like tics, fleas and mosquitoes
- Cures ear infections
- Improves digestion
- Encourages healthy and shiny fur and hair
- Maintains healthy weight
- Removes urine odor (especially in cats)

19. SIDE EFFECTS OF ACV

This is one of the common questions I get – what about any side-effects of apple cider vinegar? Apple cider vinegar is a natural product and has no known side effects, unlike many drugs in the market. Apple cider vinegar has been used in the kitchen and in our diet for centuries, and has been man's companion on rough sea voyages to unknown land. Undiluted apple cider vinegar, in liquid or pill form, may damage the esophagus (food pipe), and other parts of the digestive tract. Apple cider vinegar drinks may damage tooth enamel if sipped over a long period of time.

One health expert believes that over-consumption of cider vinegar may lower potassium level. One case report linked excessive apple cider vinegar consumption with low blood potassium levels (hypokalemia) and low bone mineral density, according to Cathy Wong,[14] ND, a naturopathic doctor, author and an American College of Nutrition-certified nutrition specialist.

This is why patients suffering from osteoporosis, low potassium levels, and those taking potassium-lowering medications must consult a doctor.

If you are allergic to apples, avoid cider vinegar.

ACV lowers blood glucose and insulin levels, and as such, people on medication for diabetes should consult a doctor, as ACV may have an additive effect and cause glucose levels to drop too low.

Similarly, ACV lowers blood pressure, and may cause blood pressure to drop dramatically in people already on medication for high blood pressure.

To get the most benefit from cider vinegar, these are some of the things to keep in mind while using it:

- Among those drinking apple cider vinegar daily, a common symptom is frequent urination. Visits to toilet increase. This is expected, with the increased amount of water consumption through the ACV drink. Also, ACV sets in motion the process of detoxification which removes waste from body through urination.

- Some people may experience sore throat, if sensitive to acidic drinks.

- While applying ACV toner on skin to remove acne, warts, pimples or generally for better skin, some people may experience skin irritation in rare cases. This could be because of two reasons: body is throwing out impurities that were clogging the openings in skin. This can cause 'breaking out', which is a normal reaction. If it persists, discontinue the application, or use ACV toner in a more diluted form, and less frequently. Second cause could be sensitivity of skin. Some people may find that their skin is not suitable for the use of ACV. In this case, discontinue it.

• Many people are concerned about the possible damage to teeth. Apple cider vinegar contains 5% acidity, which is low, and it is further diluted with water before drinking. This ensures that there is likely to be no damage to the enamel of our teeth. However, as an additional precaution, use a straw to drink ACV. This is a common practice.

• Additionally, rinse mouth with baking soda mixed in water, so that it removes any ACV left in mouth. Baking soda also helps in whitening teeth. Follow it up by rinsing with normal water to remove the residue of baking soda too.

• When applying on skin, the odor of ACV may seem too strong. For this reason, avoid using ACV on skin before going out. The best time to apply ACV toner is before going to bed.

• Limited legislation exists for regulating the quality of vinegar in the United States. The US FDA website states: "No standards of identity for vinegar have been established under the Federal Food, Drug, and Cosmetic Act."[15] The FDA specifies that ACV must contain 4% acetic acid, but ACV brands in the market are rarely checked for compliance. Do your own research before choosing an ACV brand to buy.

• If ACV bottle is exposed to air, it may cause 'vinegar eels' to develop in the bottle. Secure bottle lid tightly.

20. FREQUENTLY ASKED QUESTIONS

If you have read this far, you have completed a comprehensive guide to healthy living with cider vinegar. Before you began reading this book, you may have had many questions, and I hope you have found answers to most of them.

Every day, I receive many queries from readers. This chapter is compiled from the most common questions I receive about apple cider vinegar. If you haven't already found an answer to your queries in the book, you may likely find that information in this chapter. Let us begin.

Question: Should I drink two-teaspoon apple cider vinegar with water before each meal or two-teaspoon for the whole day?

Answer: Apple cider vinegar is normally very good for you. So you may drink it as often as you wish, as long as it is diluted. However, don't go overboard and avoid drinking excessive amounts of ACV. I have found best results are achieved when you drink it on an empty stomach - once after waking up, and then an hour before each meal. Rinse mouth clean with water after drinking ACV so that the acetic acid in vinegar doesn't get a chance to ruin the enamel on teeth. Better still, brush teeth after drinking ACV.

Question: I am just 25 years old and am trying to get pregnant after my weight loss. Will consumption of apple cider vinegar regularly have any side effects. Kindly advise.

Answer: Apple cider vinegar contains potassium which is essential for many body-functions. Being a mineral, potassium maintains electrolyte balance and release energy from fat, carbohydrates and protein. It improves digestion, and aids in the absorption of nutrients from the food we eat. As such apple cider vinegar is very good in preparing your body for a healthy pregnancy. However, once you are pregnant, you should consult your doctor before popping anything in your mouth, including apple cider vinegar.

Question: I gained 16 pounds during pregnancy, and I haven't lost any of that excess weight after delivery. I am currently breast-feeding my three-month old daughter. Can I drink cider vinegar for losing weight?

Answer: Apple cider vinegar is effective in increasing metabolism rate and assisting in burning excess fat. However, breast-feeding women should consult a doctor before introducing cider vinegar in their diet, irrespective of whether they were an ACV drinker before pregnancy.

Question: If I drink it two times a day how much weight can I lose in a week?

Answer: This is one of the most common questions I get - how fast can I lose weight with cider vinegar? Apple cider vinegar or any natural weight-loss solution may not provide overnight success. ACV works inside out, and creates a healthy gut that can burn fat, absorb nutrients and remove toxins. Each person's body as well as lifestyle is different, which can cause results to vary. ACV alone cannot cause considerable weight loss. Cider vinegar must be supported by balanced and healthy diet, and regular exercise.

It may take weeks before you notice any significant signs of weight loss. However, you will begin to feel better and more energetic right from the day you start drinking cider vinegar.

Question: Can it work if I drink cider vinegar with spinach? And is it true if I drink grapefruit juice with ACV, that can help lose weight faster?

Answer: Drink cider vinegar with grapefruit juice or orange juice to get greater health benefits. It is preferable to use fresh juice, instead of commercial juice that is usually loaded with sugar and preservatives. Also, drink fresh juice within half an hour of making it so as to get the most nutritional value out of the juice. However, it is not known whether ACV and grapefruit juice provides greater weight-loss benefits than ACV drink alone.

Spinach is loaded with fiber and vitamin C, and makes for a healthy diet. In fact, spinach contains one of the highest amounts of fiber per serving. It also provides niacin, zinc, protein, vitamins, calcium, iron and magnesium.

Question: I have lost 2 kgs in three weeks. The weight has come straight off my belly. I am less ravenous and I am eating more salads. Before the apple cider vinegar diet, I was always hungry and it felt like I was fighting my physiology by not eating huge meals. I drink it through a straw and rinse with salty water afterwards to buffer the acid to protect teeth.

I am not sure how long to take it. I think I may cut down to every second day after awhile and just monitor my calorie intake.

Answer: I am glad to know that you have managed to lose weight in three weeks. When supported by healthy diet, ACV can show miraculous results. You should continue to take cider vinegar even after achieving your weight loss goal. ACV is not just good for burning fat, but is also useful in complete well-being, as I have discussed in this book.

Question: I put two-teaspoon ACV in a 16 oz water bottle. Should I drink it all or half?

Answer: Drink only half at a time. I would start will smaller quantity to drink. Once your body has adjusted to smaller doses, you can gradually increase it. I found it useful to begin with just 8 oz (one cup) water and one-teaspoon cider vinegar.

Question: I eat junk food for lunch almost every day (except for the week-ends) because I'm a college student with no time to cook for lunch; I study from 8am to 4pm. I started drinking apple cider vinegar yesterday. What do you think? Please help me; I really need to lose weight.

Answer: While apple cider vinegar is great for weight loss, I doubt if it will help much if you are consuming a lot of junk food at the same time. Busy schedules make it difficult to follow a good diet, but a little bit of creativity can solve the problem.

Look on the Internet for cider vinegar salad recipes. You don't need to make a salad every day. Prepare salads for the whole week once and store them separately in glass jars in refrigerator. Cider vinegar acts as a good preservative. Take one salad with you to work every day.

Also don't forget to exercise at least three times a week, even if it is a 15-minute walk. Finally, make apples, spinach and broccoli a part of your daily diet - this should give you plenty of dietary fiber and other nutrients.

Question: When I drink ACV my blood sugar goes down, I feel dizzy. What should I do?

Answer: You can re-balance your blood sugar by eating baked potatoes. Baking converts the starch into blood sugar. It is a healthy snack. Also, consult your doctor if this is an ongoing issue, or if you are on any diabetes-related medication.

Question: Does apple cider vinegar help with joints? My bones are hurting all the time. Will ACV help?

Answer: Yes, apple cider vinegar is effective in reducing joint pain. Put one cup of cider vinegar in warm bath water and soak yourself in it for half an hour. Gently massage aching joints, beginning with feet and moving upwards. Feel the stress leaving your body as you work each joint softly. Keep your eyes away from the water. It is OK to soak in your hair in the bath water.

Also, apple cider vinegar is known to help in reducing weight. And with leaner body, bones and joints will have less of a reason to complain.

Question: I have a couple of questions. I am currently consuming a beetroot, apple and carrot juice in the morning on an empty stomach, and was thinking of adding a tablespoon of ACV to the juice or should it be diluted only in water? Also I am breastfeeding, and was wondering if there is any research into ACV helping with milk production?

Answer: Beetroot, apple and carrot is a great combination for fruit juice, and it's my favorite drink. I add a bit of ginger to it. And of course, you can mix a tablespoon of cider vinegar to your juice. Drink freshly-made juice as soon as it is made so as to get the most benefit from it. If you are pregnant or breastfeeding, please consult your doctor.

Question: Can cider vinegar cure acid reflux?

Answer: Yes, cider vinegar, as an acetic acid drink, is effective in preventing as well as addressing heartburn. One of my readers used to spend $75 a month on OTC drugs for acid reflux; she switched to ACV two years back, and hasn't had an 'episode' since. Take one- to three-teaspoon of cider vinegar mixed in a cup of water on an empty stomach every day, and you will be free of heartburn.

Question: I don't like the pungent taste of cider vinegar. How do I drink it?

Answer: I have found that mixing cider vinegar in lukewarm water can help you in getting over the smell as well as taste. However, please don't warm it too much, as it may alter the properties of apple cider vinegar. Some of my readers add ice to their drink with similar effect. You may also mix honey with ACV drink.

Question: Can I take the vinegar in my black tea as the taste is too much to bear? Does it counter its results? Please advise.

Answer: You may add cider vinegar to black tea if it helps in getting over the taste. However, hot water may reduce the effectiveness of cider vinegar, while caffeine in tea may interfere with the process of absorption. Try mixing ACV in fresh juice instead. Also avoid putting milk or other dairy products in an ACV drink.

Question: I am just starting to take ACV for several reasons - weight loss, sinus problems etc. I have been taking small amounts to build up to two-teaspoon to three-teaspoon before each meal. So far I feel great! It's been a great afternoon energy booster. Will mixing ACV with carbonated flavored water or EmergenC supplement packets give me all the same benefits?

Answer: The idea of diluting ACV in water is to help reduce the effect of fruit acid in the ACV, and as such, water is the best diluter. However, I don't think it should be a problem to mix it with EmergenC. I don't recommend carbonated drinks because of their adverse health effect.

Question: I am a diabetic and I take regular medicines for diabetes. Please let me know if there are any side effects of drinking cider vinegar.

Answer: ACV is made from fruits as the name suggests. As such, it contains fruit-sugar, which is not known to cause any issue for people with diabetes. In fact, ACV has positive effect on blood-sugar levels, according to WebMD. As per a 2007 study of 11 people with Type-2 diabetes, two-teaspoon of apple cider vinegar taken before bed lowers glucose levels in the morning by 4% to 6%. Since you are already on medication for diabetes, please consult your doctor so that your blood sugar doesn't drop too much.

Question: I make a concentrate - 50:50 ACV and raw honey. It needs serious shaking to blend together.

Then I put an inch of the concentrate in the bottom of my glass water bottle and fill with warm water. I finish one bottle a day. I was doing this for my overall health, as weight is not really an issue, but I have lost three pounds in 10 days. I hope this will level off soon, but I do feel great.

Answer: Because cider vinegar helps in removing toxins, and improving digestion, weight loss is normal even if that's not your goal. You are feeling more energetic with cider vinegar, which is a sign of better health.

Question: I've been taking two-teaspoon of ACV mixed with about 4 oz of orange juice in the morning after eating breakfast. Is this okay to do every day? Should I be taking more for weight loss? What about damage to my teeth? Is there a big difference in weight loss by taking more than that a day?

Answer: Ideally, drink cider vinegar first thing in the morning and an hour before a meal. Also, dilute it with 8 oz of water/juice, especially if it is an orange juice, since the juice is acetic. This will prevent any damage to your teeth. You may also choose to drink it with a straw, so as to protect your teeth, or rinse mouth with water after drinking ACV. Regarding how often one should drink, 2 to 3 times a day is ideal.

Question: I bought a regular brand of cider vinegar. Can this work or does it have to be organic?

Answer: Apple cider vinegar should be unfiltered and unpasteurized. If packaging/label on the bottle doesn't specify, it is unlikely that the vinegar is unfiltered and unpasteurized. So make sure you pick up the right vinegar. If it is also organic, that's an icing on the cake since it is certified to be free from pesticides and chemicals.

Question: I get severe stomach cramps during 'that' time of the month. Can apple cider vinegar be used to treat period pain?

Answer: Apple cider vinegar can help to reduce menstrual cramps. Drinking ACV regularly helps in regulating blood clotting and reduces the duration of period. It is reported that ACV also reduces the amount of blood that you lose, and in turn helps prevent anemia.

When applied externally, ACV can also relieve menstrual pain. Dampen a cloth in warm water mixed with a quarter cup of ACV and put it on stomach. Cover the cloth with a hot water bottle. Leave it on for 20 minutes. This should relieve the stomach pain.

Question: I have thyroid problem for many years. Does ACV help with thyroids?

Answer: You haven't mentioned whether you are enquiring about hyperthyroid or hypothyroid. In any case, there's little medical advice that confirms the usefulness of ACV in treating thyroid problems. However, cider vinegar is known to regulate hormones and improve metabolism. This may provide rest to thyroid and improve its function.

In the absence of research-based evidence, you will need to see what works best for you. Try cider vinegar for a few days (one-teaspoon to three-teaspoon a day) and then take the thyroid test. If your reports show improvement, then you know that cider vinegar has been effective.

Where little research exists to support the usefulness of cider vinegar for a particular illness, it helps to remember that ACV supports overall health since it is a fermented drink. Fermentation helps in breaking down proteins into amino acids, which are absolutely essential for a healthy body. Amino acids carry and store nutrients. They are also essential for good metabolism.

The enzymes in vinegar help in building good flora in stomach. All these factors help in creating a stronger immune system, which in turn makes it possible to fight many illnesses.

Question: I'm wondering if I can get the same benefits that ACV offers in pill form - 500mg, three times daily? I have a very difficult time drinking it, even diluted as suggested.

Answer: Let us look at a research entitled "*Therapeutic Effect Of Daily Vinegar Ingestion For Individuals At Risk For Type 2 Diabetes*" conducted by Carol S. Johnston, Samantha Quagliano, and Serena Whit from School of Nutrition and Health Promotion, Arizona State University (quoted earlier in this book).

The study recommended using apple cider vinegar drink instead of pills. Researchers noted: "Commercial vinegar tablets do not contain adequate amounts of acetic acid to induce an antiglycemic effect." Remember, this research was specifically in relation to diabetes. If you are unable to drink cider vinegar and have to take it in tablet form, please consult a good pharmacist.

Question: I am thinking of losing weight with Dinintel tabs. Can I take these tabs while I am drinking ACV?

Answer: Dinintel contains the active ingredient clobenzorex, which is a stimulant used as an appetite suppressant. Cider vinegar helps in improving metabolism. These two foods have different approaches, and may or may not go well together for some people. Please consult a doctor.

Question: I usually drink ACV with cold water. Can it be consumed with hot water and if yes, how?

Answer: Avoid mixing ACV with hot water as it may reduce the effectiveness of enzymes. It is best to mix it with lukewarm water so that it is easy on your throat. You can mix it with honey to make it more palatable. And honey has many health benefits too.

Question: I am 14 and suffering from obesity. How much time will it take for ACV to help me lose weight?

Answer: Losing weight with apple cider vinegar is a marathon, not sprint. So give it some time. Also, review your diet to make sure you are not eating any junk. You can compliment ACV with regular exercise.

Question: Is it better to mix one-teaspoon ACV in 1 cup orange juice with one-teaspoon honey, or in one cup warm water with one-teaspoon honey?

Answer: My preference would be honey and water. This is because orange juice already has acidic content, which may add to ACV's acidity. It terms of health benefits, it shouldn't make a difference, except the unnecessary consumption of sugar contained in commercial orange juices. Use fresh juice where possible.

Question: I want to put ACV drink in a plastic bottle and take it with me. Will it break down the plastic in bottles it is mixed in? I have it sitting on my desk so I remember to finish it. I don't want to drink plastic if it breaks down into the mixture. Should I be mixing it in glass jars instead?

Answer: Most plastic bottles that are meant to carry food and drink are made from polyethylene terephthalate (PET). The PET bottles are approved by the United States FDA (1998) for food storage. The 5% acetic acid contained in cider vinegar will have minor impact on plastic, that too in the long run. If it is for daily use, you can carry your ACV drink in PET bottles. Just to be safe, store the bottle away from sun light, in a cool place. For long-term storage (more than a few months), use glass jars. This is the reason I buy cider vinegar that's packaged in a glass bottle. Remember, apple cider vinegar doesn't have an expiry date.

Question: Can I consume ACV immediately in the morning after I get up and then have tea and leave for

work and have lunch in office straight at 1.30pm? I usually don't have breakfast. And can I mix it with lemon juice and water?

Answer: Yes, ideally ACV should be consumed on an empty stomach. However, it is advisable to have breakfast, as it gives a head-start to a hectic day. It is easier to digest food early in the day, and as such, you can get away with eating junk food if it is consumed at the beginning of the day.

Heavy breakfast also means you will eat smaller meals later in the day, which is ideal if you are trying to stay healthy. Eating a big breakfast of 700 calories promotes weight loss and reduces risks for diabetes, heart disease and high cholesterol, according to a study conducted by Tel Aviv University professor, Daniela Jakubowicz, published in the *Obesity*.[16]

To answer your second question, many people mix ACV with honey and/or lemon juice and water, which makes a nice drink.

Question: I have read that cider vinegar erodes the enamel on teeth. Is this true?

Answer: The outer layer of our teeth is called enamel, with is made of calcium mineral. The acetic acid in vinegar has a demineralizing effect on teeth - that is - it erodes the calcium and sets in motion the process of tooth decay. Which is why you should always take following precautions to prevent tooth decay:

- Dilute cider vinegar with water
- Use a straw to drink ACV
- If you haven't used a straw, brush teeth after drinking cider vinegar
- Alternatively, rinse mouth with water after drinking ACV. For more protection, add baking soda to water and rinse. Follow this rinse with a water rinse.

Question: I have been using ACV for about a month, taking 1 tablespoon before meals. I liked it at first; but it has started making me feel sick. Why is this? Should I continue to take it?

Answer: Apple cider vinegar is natural fruit drink if it is organic, and rarely has side effects. If it is making you sick, discontinue it for a while and see how you feel. You may try again after some time.

Question: I am drinking ACV for the past three days - adding two-teaspoon in a glass and mixing it with water only. I don't feel any heartburn now. I am worried about long-term effects of drinking cider vinegar.

Answer: There are no known side effects of apple cider vinegar. Drinking cider vinegar is safe. Many people have shared their positive experiences of losing weight with apple cider vinegar. It is very effective for other ailments too. However, you may want to take periodic breaks from drinking cider vinegar, so that your body doesn't get too dependent on it. I would suggest taking a week-long break every two months or so and notice how you feel.

Question: My husband has constipation problem for so long. We have tried many things; but nothing has worked so far. Will ACV work in his case, and how long does he need to take it?

Answer: Apple cider vinegar is great for improving digestion. If your husband is currently constipated, then ACV may not be an immediate solution. You may want to administer some laxative from the pharmacy. Once motions are back to normal, start drinking cider vinegar every day to keep the stomach in good digestive state.

Question: I have been drinking ACV for seven weeks now, and I feel great. However, I visit the bathroom a lot. Is this normal?

Answer: Since you are mixing ACV with water, you are drinking more water than you would normally do. As such, you are urinating more frequently. Also, ACV is removing toxins from the body, which may cause more urination.

Question: I know ACV is supposed to curb my appetite and sometimes it does. At times I feel really full, but at other times I just cant seem to stop eating because I stay hungry. What should I do?

Answer: Cider vinegar is not likely to suppress your appetite. It increases your metabolism and removes toxins, making your digestion system healthier. As a result, you may feel hungry more often. Make sure you are eating and drinking healthy food.

Question: I am trying out ACV. However I read

that we must keep our bodies in an alkaline state and therefore I am also drinking alkaline water. So does drinking the acidic ACV nullify the effect of alkalinity of our bodies?

Answer: I can give a long answer. However, let's keep this brief. Human body is an amazing mechanism, and it maintains a good balance despite varied foods and drinks we consume, with varied acidic and alkali content. This is called Homeostasis. As such, drinking alkaline water and ACV should be okay. Whether alkaline water is of any benefit to human health is a topic of debate currently.

Question: What is your opinion about mixing honey, cinnamon and cayenne pepper in cider vinegar drink?

Answer: Mixing honey in ACV is common. Adding cinnamon is also popular as it helps to further speed up metabolism. Adding cayenne pepper maybe an option if it doesn't make cider vinegar drink too spicy. All this will help boost metabolism.

Question: Will cider vinegar bloat my stomach?

Answer: No, cider vinegar will not bloat stomach. To the contrary, cider vinegar will assist digestion system in processing food better, and you will experience smoother bowel movement, and healthy stomach.

Question: My 14-year daughter is drinking ACV behind my back. Is it good for her age?

Answer: ACV is a natural product, and if it is made from organic apples, that will be icing on the cake. It should be OK for your 14-year old daughter, as long as she sticks to the prescribed limit. She will get lots of health benefits from drinking ACV, and it's better than drinking caffeine-based or aerated drinks. Please make sure she drinks it diluted and rinses mouth after drinking it.

Question: I'm using an ACV tablet from Sweden. The strength is 600 mg. If I switch to liquid form, how long can I take it for and in what quantity?

Answer: If you switch to liquid ACV, you can take it for lifetime. It's a natural product. Apple cider vinegar is made from organic apples and has no known side effects. You can take it twice a day - mid-morning and mid-evening, before meals. You will feel renewed energy and better digestion.

Question: My mother has cancer of the stomach (gastric cancer). Can she take ACV?

Answer: while there isn't sufficient evidence to support any claim of ACV's use for stomach cancer, it wouldn't hurt to try ACV for your mother. ACV is known to improve digestion and remove toxins from the stomach. However, since she may already be on medication, please consult a good doctor.

Question: Can I drink ACV after my meal?

Answer: Ideally, you should drink ACV before meals. This helps in improving the performance of the digestion system, which is essential for removing toxins.

Question: Is it okay to put pure ACV directly on a cotton ball and leave it on my ringworm overnight?

Answer: It is advisable to try leaving ACV on your ringworm for about 15 minutes first and see if it results in any reaction. If it doesn't, then you should be OK to leave it on overnight. Also make sure that apple cider vinegar remains limited to the ringworm area, and doesn't come in contact with healthy skin as this may cause skin irritation in some people.

Question: I take diet pills. Is it okay to take my diet pill with cider vinegar water? If not, how long should I wait before I can take my diet pills after drinking ACV water?

Answer: A variety of diet pills are available in the market, which work differently. As such, it is difficult to advise. Please consult your doctor.

Question: I read that ACV helps with bad breath or halitosis. I read that I should mix ACV with water and gargle with it. After the gargle, do I need to rinse out with regular water to prevent damaging my enamel?

Answer: Yes, cider vinegar is effective in preventing bad breath. You can use it as a mouthwash. Put one-teaspoon cider vinegar in a cup of water and rinse your mouth with it. It helps in preventing gum disease, killing harmful bacteria, and removing plaque and tartar. It is advisable to rinse with water after ACV rinse.

Question: If I have ulcers will this bother or irritate ulcers?

Answer: If you have any medical condition, including ulcers, you must consult your physician before starting the apple cider vinegar diet.

Question: I am a college student with hypothyroidism. I would gain weight from eating anything, even if it were healthy. I recently started drinking ACV around three weeks ago and lately I have not been able to follow my strict diet. But I'm not gaining any weight at all. In fact I've been looking slimmer! I was wondering if it would be feasible to lose 10 lbs in the next 3.5 months followed with an average/not unhealthy diet.

Answer: People with hypothyroidism are likely to benefit from apple cider vinegar diet. ACV helps in regulating metabolism, which in turn gives rest to thyroid gland.

Increased metabolism is useful for people with hypothyroidism who are keen to lose weight. Yes, it is possible to lose 10 lbs in three months - which is about 3 lbs every month. Make sure you eat healthy food. I would also recommend adding a bit of physical exercise thrice a week - swimming, dancing, running, trade-mill - whatever you love doing. Cider vinegar boosts metabolism, and when you add some exercise to the routine, it multiplies the benefits of losing weight. Also, cider vinegar re-balances pH factor, thus improving digestion, and strengthening immune system. All this adds up in your efforts of shedding extra pounds.

Question: I am keen to try apple cider vinegar. Can I use commercial cider vinegar because I can't find organic ACV. Also, is it healthy to use bottled water instead of filtered water? And can I use commercial honey instead of organic honey, and lemon juice concentrate?

Answer: If you cannot find organic ACV or honey, use the regular ones. Just make sure that the ACV is unpasteurized and unfiltered. Avoid juice concentrate if you can, as it may contain preservatives. Bottled water is fine too.

Question: I love the taste of this stuff, and just drink it straight out of the bottle. I may be strange, but I wash it down with water to help my teeth. How much of this stuff would I have to drink before it became unhealthy?

Answer: Apple cider vinegar is a natural product and as such it is safe to drink. However, you wouldn't want to go overboard, as it can upset stomach. You don't want the pH balance of your stomach going haywire, especially if you are drinking it undiluted. Stick to one- to three-teaspoon per glass of water, three times a day. If you are drinking straight from the bottle, follow it up with a thorough mouth rinse with water.

Question: Can I give ACV to my 6-year old son?

Answer: There's not much evidence for or against

giving ACV to young children. My friend's daughter loves ACV with honey. She is 12. You may start with a very small quantity (a couple of ACV drops in a cup of water and one-teaspoon honey), and see how you go. Please make sure that your son sticks to the prescribed limit, and rinses mouth after drinking ACV.

Question: I am taking honey cinnamon with warm water first thing in the morning and last thing before going to bed. Is it okay to take honey cinnamon and then ACV, followed by breakfast?

Answer: Yes, that sounds like a good plan. Or mix honey and cinnamon with ACV and drink before breakfast. Try to keep half an hour's break between ACV drink and breakfast.

Question: Could the mixture of honey, cinnamon and ACV stay outdoors for four to five hours? I'm working and want to take this drink with me to workplace.

Answer: Yes, your ACV drink should remain fresh outdoors. Cider vinegar has preservative qualities and can stay in good condition at room temperature. Avoid storing it in direct sunlight.

Question: I have problematic oily skin with acne or pimples. Will drinking ACV work for it, or do I need to apply it to the face too?

Answer: Yes, drinking ACV improves digestion and overall wellbeing. So it will help with your issue of oily skin. This is because good health is reflected in healthy skin. In addition, you can apply ACV toner on your skin before going to bed.

EPILOGUE

Apples are a nature's gift to us - to help us lead a fuller life. Apple cider vinegar goes through a fermentation process which adds to the amazing qualities of apples.

Making apple cider vinegar a part of diet is a conscious choice. It is the first step towards taking control of wellbeing.

However, leading a healthy life is not limited to drinking cider vinegar twice a day. It is a beginning. Vinegar prepares body for a good living.

We must complement it with regular exercise, stress management through meditation, healthy diet, and vitamins and mineral supplements.

It is only when we take the ownership of our well-being and make a commitment for wholesome living that we begin our journey towards a disease-free life.

BEFORE YOU GO

I hope you enjoyed reading this book, and found valuable tips for improving your health.

I believe that each of us has the ability to lead a healthy life, and I am positive that this book has provided you with ideas for improving your health.

Thank you for reading this book. I would like to hear from you. Please take a moment to write a review on Amazon. I read all reviews of my book; it's the real reward for writing this book.

I will leave you with a link to my website, where you can access free health articles and resources, and send me your queries:

Visit: www.101WaysToLife.com.

DISCLAIMER

The contents of this book are for informational purposes only and not intended to be a substitute for professional medical advice, diagnosis or treatment. Always seek the advice of your physician or other qualified health provider with any questions you may have regarding a medical condition. Never disregard professional medical advice or delay in seeking it on account of the contents of this book.

If you have a medical emergency, call your doctor immediately. Reliance on any information provided in this book is solely at your own risk. The author and publisher of this book are not liable for any loss or damage arising out of the use of information contained in this book.

ABOUT THE AUTHOR

V. Gangan is an international journalist and editor, with two decades of writing and publishing experience. He is passionate about complementary medicine and wellbeing. He lives in green and beautiful New Zealand.

REFERENCES

[1] Koutsos, A., & Lovegrove, J. (2014). An Apple a Day Keeps the Doctor Away – Inter-Relationship Between Apple Consumption, the Gut Microbiota and Cardiometabolic Disease Risk Reduction. Diet-Microbe Interactions In The Gut, 173-194. doi:10.1016/b978-0-12-407825-3.00012-5

[2] Shoji, T., & Miura, T. (2014). Apple Polyphenols in Cancer Prevention. Polyphenols In Human Health And Disease, 1373-1383. doi:10.1016/b978-0-12-398456-2.00104-3

[3] Bhagwat, S., Haytowitz, D., & Holden, J. (2007). USDA database for the Oxygen Radical Absorbance Capacity (ORAC) of selected foods, 1--2

[4] Bongers, A., Risse, L., & Bus, V. (1993). Physical and Chemical Characteristics of Apples From Several Countries. Hortscience, 28(5), 446-446. Retrieved from http://hortsci.ashspublications.org/content/28/5/446.5.abstract

[5] Herper, M. (2013). The Cost Of Creating A New Drug Now $5 Billion. Forbes. Retrieved 20 August 2014, from http://www.forbes.com/sites/matthewherper/2013/08/11/how-the-staggering-cost-of-inventing-new-drugs-is-shaping-the-future-of-medicine/

[6] Lazarou, J., Pomeranz, B., & Corey, P. (1998). Incidence of adverse drug reactions in hospitalized patients: a meta-analysis of prospective studies. Jama, 279(15), 1200—1205

[7] Authors: Tomoo Kondo, Mikiya Kishi, Takashi Fushimi, Shinobu Ugajin, and Takayuki Kaga, Central Research Institute, Mizkan Group Corporation. Published: Bioscience, Biotechnology, and Biochemistry Vol. 73 (2009) No. 8 P 1837-1843, released 23 August 2009

[8] Department of Nutrition, Para-Medical School, Ahvaz Jundishapour

University of Medical Sciences, Ahvaz, Islamic Republic of Iran.
Pakistan Journal of Biological Sciences 12/2008; 11(23):2634-8

[9] The FASEB Journal. 2013;27:1079.56

[10] http://www.aad.org/media-resources/stats-and-facts/conditions/psoriasis

[11] Earthclinic.com,. (2014). Varicose Vein Treatment: Home Cures.
Retrieved 10 August 2014, from
http://www.earthclinic.com/cures/varicose-vein-treatment-natural-remedies.html

[12] Webmd.com,. (2014). Varicose Veins Causes, Symptoms, and
Treatments. Retrieved 17 August 2014, from
http://www.webmd.com/skin-problems-and-treatments/tc/varicose-veins-topic-overview

[13] Bragg, P., & Bragg, P. (n.d.). Apple Cider Vinegar Miracle Health
System (1st ed.). Santa Barbara, Calif.: Health Science

[14] Cathy Wong, N. (2014). The Health Benefits of Apple Cider
Vinegar. About.com Alternative Medicine. Retrieved 20 August
2014, from
http://altmedicine.about.com/od/applecidervinegardiet/a/applecid
ervineg.htm

[15] Fda.gov, (2014). CPG Sec. 525.825 Vinegar, Definitions -
Adulteration with Vinegar Eels. [online] Available at:
http://www.fda.gov/iceci/compliancemanuals/compliancepolicygui
dancemanual/ucm074471.htm [Accessed 11 Sep. 2014].

[16] Jakubowicz, D., Barnea, M., Wainstein, J. and Froy, O. (2013), High
Caloric intake at breakfast vs. dinner differentially influences weight
loss of overweight and obese women. Obesity, 21: 2504–2512. doi:
10.1002/oby.20460

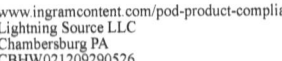